Oxford Case Histories in TIA and Stroke

HARVEY

Oxford Case Histories

Series Editors

Sarah Pendlebury and Peter Rothwell

Published:

Neurological Case Histories (Sarah Pendlebury, Philip Anslow, and Peter Rothwell)

Oxford Case Histories in Cardiology (Rajkumar Rajendram, Javed Ehtisham, and Colin Forfar)

Oxford Case Histories in Gastroenterology and Hepatology (Alissa Walsh, Otto Buchel, Jane Collier, and Simon Travis)

Oxford Case Histories in Respiratory Medicine (John Stradling, Andrew Stanton, Anabell Nickol, Helen Davies, and Najib Rahman)

Oxford Case Histories in Rheumatology (Joel David, Anne Miller, Anushka Soni, and Lyn Williamson)

Oxford Case Histories in TIA and Stroke (Sarah Pendlebury, Ursula Schulz, Aneil Malhotra, and Peter Rothwell)

Forthcoming:

Oxford Case Histories in Neurosurgery (Harutomo Hasegawa, Matthew Crocker, and Pawanjit Singh Minhas)

Oxford Case Histories in Geriatrics (Sanja Thompson, Nicola Lovett, Sarah Pendlebury, and John Grimley Evans)

Oxford Case Histories in TIA and Stroke

Sarah Pendlebury
Consultant Physician,
NIHR Biomedical Research Centre,
Research Fellow, Stroke Prevention Research Unit
Nuffield Department of Clinical Neurosciences
John Radcliffe Hospital
Oxford, UK

Ursula Schulz
NIHR Clinician Scientist and Honorary Consultant Neurologist
Stroke Prevention Research Unit
Nuffield Department of Clinical Neurosciences
John Radcliffe Hospital
University Department of Clinical Neurology
Oxford, UK

Aneil Malhotra
Cardiology Specialist Registrar
John Radcliffe Hospital
Oxford Deanery
Oxford, UK

Peter M. Rothwell
Director, Stroke Prevention Research Unit,
Nuffield Department of Clinical Neurosciences
John Radcliffe Hospital
Professor of Clinical Neurology, University of Oxford,
Oxford, UK

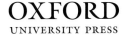

OXFORD
UNIVERSITY PRESS

OXFORD

UNIVERSITY PRESS

Great Clarendon Street, Oxford ox2 6dp

Oxford University Press is a department of the University of Oxford.
It furthers the University's objective of excellence in research, scholarship,
and education by publishing worldwide in

Oxford New York

Auckland Cape Town Dar es Salaam Hong Kong Karachi
Kuala Lumpur Madrid Melbourne Mexico City Nairobi
New Delhi Shanghai Taipei Toronto

With offices in

Argentina Austria Brazil Chile Czech Republic France Greece
Guatemala Hungary Italy Japan Poland Portugal Singapore
South Korea Switzerland Thailand Turkey Ukraine Vietnam

Oxford is a registered trade mark of Oxford University Press
in the UK and in certain other countries

Published in the United States
by Oxford University Press Inc., New York

British Library Cataloguing in Publication Data
Data available

Library of Congress Cataloging in Publication Data
Library of Congress Control Number: 2011945386

Typeset in Minion by Cenveo, Bangalore, India
Printed in Great Britain
on acid-free paper by
CPI Group (UK) Ltd, Croydon, CR0 4YY

ISBN 978–0–19–953934–5

10 9 8 7 6 5 4 3 2 1

A note from the series editors

Case histories have always had an important role in medical education, but most published material has been directed at undergraduates or residents. The Oxford Case Histories series aims to provide more complex case-based learning for clinicians in specialist training and consultants, with a view to aiding preparation for entry- and exit-level specialty examinations or revalidation.

Each case book follows the same format with approximately 50 cases, each comprising a brief clinical history and investigations, followed by questions on differential diagnosis and management, and detailed answers with discussion.

All cases are peer-reviewed by Oxford consultants in the relevant specialty. At the end of each book, cases are listed by mode of presentation, aetiology, and diagnosis. We are grateful to our colleagues in the various medical specialties for their enthusiasm and hard work in making the series possible.

Sarah Pendlebury and Peter Rothwell

From reviews of other books in the series:

Neurological Case Histories
'. . . contains 51 cases that cover the spectrum of acute neurology and the neurology of general medicine—this breadth makes the volume unique and provides a formidable challenge . . . it is a heavy-duty diagnostic series of cases, and readers have to work hard, to recognise the diagnosis and answer the questions that are posed for each case . . . I recommend this excellent volume highly. . .'
Lancet Neurology

This short and well-written text is . . . designed to enhance the reader's diagnostic ability and clinical understanding . . . A well-documented and practical book.'
European Journal of Neurology

Oxford Case Histories in Gastroenterology and Hepatology
'. . . a fascinating insight in to clinical gastroenterology, an excellent and enjoyable read and an education for all levels of gastroenterologist from ST1 to consultant.'
Gut

Preface

The profile of stroke medicine has grown enormously in recent years owing to developments in neuroimaging and treatments which have been accompanied by a rise in stroke-related research and thus knowledge about the condition. Stroke medicine is now an accepted specialty in its own right, spanning acute medicine, neurology, geriatrics, and rehabilitation medicine.

Our aim in writing this book was to collect together a series of cases of interest and educational value to stroke physicians and those in general internal and emergency medicine, geriatrics, and neurology that would illustrate the breadth and complexity of stroke. The cases cover common and uncommon causes of stroke, management dilemmas, and conditions that may mimic cerebrovascular events.

The format follows that of the other books in this series: case reports with questions followed by answers including detailed discussion of the diagnosis, differential diagnoses where relevant, and treatment. This format was chosen because it is extremely difficult to illustrate the practical process of clinical management within the traditional textbook format and the best way to learn is through analysis of individual cases. Also, we believe it is more interesting to consider real cases, and one's own differential diagnosis and treatment, than to read a text which does not require any effort on the part of the reader.

A quick note for non-UK readers: in the United Kingdom, patients with TIA or minor stroke are often managed as outpatients. They are assessed in dedicated 'TIA clinics'. These clinics are perhaps somewhat inaccurately called TIA clinics, even though both patients with TIA and with mild stroke are seen. We have also used this terminology in our book, as it reflects our clinical practice.

We would like to thank the following general physicians, stroke physicians, neurologists, and cardiologists for contributing cases, images, and/or for helpful comments on the manuscript: Dr William Bradlow, Dr Florim Cuculi, Dr Dennis Briley, Dr Matthew Giles, Dr Maggie Hammersley, Dr Hywel Jones, Dr Nicola Jones, Dr George Pope, Dr Sarah Smith, Dr Sanja Thompson, and Dr Andy Walden. Particular thanks go to Dr Wilhelm Küker for help with the neuroradiology and to Mrs Jean Brooks for secretarial assistance.

Sarah Pendlebury
Ursula Schulz
Aneil Malhotra
Peter Rothwell
Oxford 2011

Contents

Abbreviations

μ	micro
ACA	anterior cerebral artery
ACE	angiotensin-converting enzyme
ACE-R	Addenbrooke's Cognitive Examination Revised
AD	Alzheimer's disease
ADC	apparent diffusion coefficient
ADEM	acute demyelinating encephalomyelitis
AF	atrial fibrillation
AlkP	alkaline phosphatase
ALS	amyotrophic lateral sclerosis
ALT	alanine aminotransferase
ANCA	antineutrophil cytoplasmic antibody
ANF	antinuclear factor
AP	anteroposterior
APB	atrial premature beat
APTT	activated partial thromboplastin time
ASA	atrial septal aneurysm
ASD	atrial septal defect
AVM	arteriovenous malformation
BBE	Bickerstaff brainstem encephalitis
BMB	brain microbleed
BMI	body mass index
Ca	calcium
CAA	cerebral amyloid angiopathy
CABG	coronary artery bypass graft
CADASIL	cerebral autosomal dominant arteriopathy with subcortical infarcts and leukoencephalopathy
CBS	cystathionine β-synthase
CE-MRA	contrast-enhanced MRA
CGT	chorionic gonadotrophin
CI	confidence interval
CJD	Creutzfeldt–Jakob disease
CN	cranial nerve
CNS	central nervous system
Cr	creatinine
CRP	C-reactive protein
CSF	cerebrospinal fluid
CT	computed tomography
CTA	CT angiography
CVST	cerebral venous sinus thrombosis
CXR	chest X-ray
DIC	disseminated intravascular coagulation
DSA	digital subtraction angiography
DSM-IV	*Diagnostic and Statistical Manual of Mental Disorders*, 4th Edition
DVLA	Driver and Vehicle Licensing Agency
DWI	diffusion-weighted imaging
ECG	electrocardiogram
EEG	electroencephalography
EFNS	European Federation of Neurological Societies
EMG	electromyography
EVD	extraventricular drain
FBC	full blood count
FLAIR	fluid-attenuated inversion recovery
FMD	fibromuscular dysplasia
fMRI	functional MRI
GCA	giant cell arteritis
GCS	Glasgow Coma Scale
GRE	gradient echo imaging
HITS	high-intensity transient signals
ICA	internal carotid artery
ICD-10	*International Statistical Classification of Diseases and Related Health Problems, 10th Revision*
ICH	intracerebral haemorrhage

IE	infective endocarditis	PA	pulmonary artery
IgG	immunoglobin G	PAF	paroxysmal atrial fibrillation
INR	international normalized ratio	PCA	posterior cerebral artery
IV	intravenous	PCR	polymerase chain reaction
IVBCL	intravascular large B-cell lymphoma	PEG	percutaneous endoscopic gastroscopy
JVP	jugular venous pressure	PFO	patent foramen ovale
K	potassium	PRES	posterior reversible encephalopathy syndrome
LDH	lactate dehydrogenase		
LFT	liver function test	PT	prothrombin time
MCA	middle cerebral artery	PTA	persistent trigeminal artery
MMSE	Mini-Mental State Examination	RCVS	reversible cerebral vasoconstriction syndrome
MND	motor neuron disease		
MoCA	Montreal Cognitive Assessment	SAH	subarachnoid haemorrhage
MRA	magnetic resonance angiography/angiogram	SDH	subdural haematoma
		SLE	systemic lupus erythematosus
MRI	magnetic resonance imaging/image	TGA	transient global amnesia
		TIA	transient ischaemic attack
mRS	modified Rankin Scale	TOE	transoesophageal echocardiogram
MS	multiple sclerosis		
MTHFR	methylene tetrahydrofolate reductase	TOF-MRA	time-of-flight MRA
		TPA	tissue plasminogen activator
NNT	number needed to treat	TTE	transthoracic echocardiogram
OR	odds ratio	VZV	varicella zoster virus
OT	occupational therapy	WCC	white cell count

Table of normal ranges

Test	Value	Unit
Haemoglobin (Hb)	12–16 (women), 13–17 (men)	g/dl
WCC	4–11	10^9/l
Neutrophils	2–7	10^9/l
Lymphocytes	1–4	10^9/l
Platelets	150–400	10^9/l
ESR	<20 (women), <14 (men)	mm/h
aPTT	26–36	sec
PT	13–16	sec
Vit B12	180–900	ng/l
Folate	4–24	µg/l
Sodium (Na)	135–145	mmol/l
Potassium (K)	3.5–5.0	mmol/l
Urea (U)	2.5–6.7	mmol/l
Creatinine (Cr)	70–150	µmol/l
Glucose	3.0–5.5 (fasting)	mmol/l
C-reactive Protein (CRP)	<8	mg/l
Bilirubin	3–17	µmol/l
ALT	10–45	iU/l
AST	15–42	iU/l
Alkaline phosphatase (Alk P)	95–320	iU/l
Albumin	35–50	g/l
γ-GT	15–40	iU/l
Creatine Kinase (CK)	24–195	iU/l
Total Cholesterol	< 5.2	mmol/l
HDL Cholesterol	0.8–1.8	mmol/l
TSH	0.35–5.5	mU/l
fT4	10.5–20	pmol/l
IgG	6.0–13.0	g/l
IgA	0.8–3.0	g/l
IgM	0.4–2.5	g/l

Test	Value	Unit
C3	65–190	mg/dl
C4	14–40	mg/dl
Anti-cardiolipin antibodies	0–15	GPL–U/ml
Cerebrospinal fluid		
WBC	<5	cells per µl
Protein	150–400	mg/l
Glucose	at least 60% of serum glucose	mmol/l
Opening pressure	7–18	cm H_2O

Case 1

Case 1.A

A 68-year-old woman awoke from sleep but had difficulty getting out of bed as she kept falling back onto her left side. When she got up she had some weakness of her left arm, hand, and foot. Her husband also noticed a left-sided facial droop and slurred speech. Her symptoms fluctuated over the course of the day before improving. Her past medical history included hypertension for which she was taking amlodipine.

The patient was reviewed by her family doctor later on the same day. He found a left-sided hemiparesis affecting her face, arm, and leg, and brisk reflexes on the left. Blood pressure was 190/90mmHg and heart rate was 84bpm in sinus rhythm. Heart sounds were normal and there were no carotid bruits. She was reviewed at the transient ischaemic attack (TIA) clinic 24 hours later, at which time her left-sided weakness had fully resolved.

Case 1.B

A 76-year-old man was sitting at his office desk when he suffered sudden onset of left arm and hand weakness and sensory loss. An hour later the sensory deficit had resolved completely but there was still significant weakness. Six hours later he was completely back to normal. There were no other neurological symptoms or headache associated with the episode. His past medical history included hypothyroidism treated with levothyroxine.

He was referred to the TIA clinic and was seen 3 days later. At this time, his blood pressure was 165/90mmHg and heart rate was 76bpm in sinus rhythm. General and neurological examination was normal.

Case 1.C

A 53-year-old man developed sudden-onset odd behaviour and walked to the shops with his shoes under his arm. His wife also noticed that he was unable to read and had word-finding difficulties. His symptoms resolved over 90 minutes. There was no significant past medical history.

On examination in the TIA clinic two days later, his blood pressure was 140/70mmHg and pulse 66bpm in sinus rhythm. He had some nominal dysphasia but the remainder of the neurological examination was normal.

Questions

1. What is the most likely diagnosis in these patients? Give a differential diagnosis for transient episodes of sudden onset focal neurological deficit.

2. What is the traditional definition of a TIA?

3. How have definitions of TIA and stroke changed recently?

4. Each patient had a CT brain performed on the day of their clinic attendance (see Figs 1.1–1.3). Describe the abnormalities on each scan.

5. The follow-up scans of Cases 1.A and 1.C are shown in Figs 1.4 and 1.5. What do you think is the most likely diagnosis now?

6. How often do patients referred to a dedicated TIA clinic turn out not to have had a cerebrovascular event?

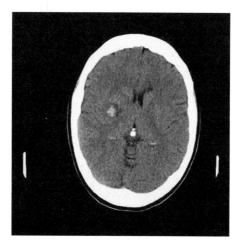

Fig. 1.1 Case 1.A: CT brain.

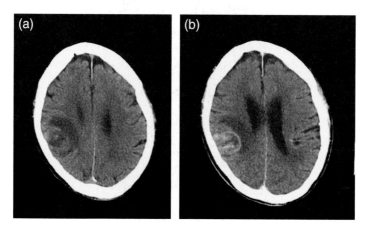

Fig. 1.2 Case 1.B: CT brain (a) without and (b) with contrast.

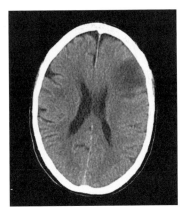

Fig. 1.3 Case 1.C: CT brain.

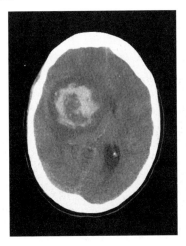

Fig. 1.4 Case 1.A 2 months after presentation: CT brain with contrast.

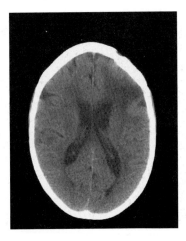

Fig. 1.5 Case 1.C 3 months after presentation: CT brain.

Answers

1. What is the most likely diagnosis in these patients? Give a differential diagnosis for transient episodes of sudden onset focal neurological deficit.

The most likely diagnosis in all three cases is TIA (minor stroke in Case 1.C), given the sudden onset of a focal neurological deficit in a middle-aged or elderly patient with vascular risk factors, resolution of the symptoms within 24 hours (also see answer to Question 2), and absence of any obvious other explanation at the time of the first clinical assessment.

While transient ischaemia is the most likely diagnosis, other conditions may also cause transient focal neurological symptoms (Table 1.1). However, there will frequently be markers in the history pointing towards the correct diagnosis. Furthermore, in some of these conditions (e.g. tumours or inflammatory lesions) longer-lasting deficits are much more common, although transient deficits may occasionally occur.

2. What is the traditional definition of a TIA?

The traditional definition of a TIA dates back to the mid-1960s. Then, a TIA was defined as 'an acute loss of focal brain or monocular function with symptoms lasting less than 24 hours, which is thought to be caused by inadequate cerebral or ocular

Table 1.1 Causes of transient focal neurological deficits

TIA
Migraine with aura (see Case 7)
Partial epileptic seizures (see Cases 6, 23, and 42)
Structural intracranial lesions
Tumour
Chronic subdural haematoma (see Case 46)
Vascular malformation (see Case 44)
Giant aneurysm (see Case 21)
Multiple sclerosis (see Case 13)
Labyrinthine disorders: Ménière's disease, or benign positional vertigo
Peripheral nerve or root lesion (see Case 26)
Metabolic
Hypoglycaemia
Hyperglycaemia
Hypercalcaemia
Hyponatraemia
Non-organic/psychogenic (see Cases 12 and 20)

blood supply as a result of arterial thrombosis, low flow or embolism associated with arterial, cardiac or haematological disease'. Stroke was defined as 'rapidly developing clinical symptoms and/or signs of focal, and at times global loss of brain function, with symptoms lasting more than 24 hours or leading to death, with no apparent cause other than that of vascular origin'. Differentiating a TIA from a stroke was thus based on symptom duration of less than versus more than 24 hours, respectively.

3. How have definitions of TIA and stroke changed recently?

Over the last decade, the definition for TIA has been challenged and revised. The 24-hour cut-off is arbitrary, as most TIAs resolve within 60 minutes. The classical definition of a TIA is purely based on clinical criteria; it does not take into account any imaging or pathological information. However, with the increasing availability of high-quality brain imaging, in particular diffusion-weighted MRI (DWI), it has become obvious that even patients with very brief neurological symptoms may have evidence of tissue infarction.

The American Stroke Association and American Heart Association have recently addressed this potential conflict between clinical and imaging findings, and they have re-defined a TIA as 'a transient episode of neurological dysfunction caused by focal brain, spinal cord, or retinal ischaemia, without acute infarction' (Easton *et al.* 2009). Stroke is defined as 'an infarction of central nervous system tissue'. There has been some debate about these new definitions, as they require brain imaging which may not always be possible, especially in less developed countries. The new definitions for TIA and stroke may be helpful in some stroke studies, especially in prognostic studies, or in studies with specific imaging inclusion criteria. However, in the future it may be more difficult to compare the findings of stroke incidence studies, as the incidence of stroke and TIA will clearly depend on which definitions are used, and on whether the diagnosis of TIA and stroke is based purely on clinical criteria or also includes imaging information.

4. Each patient had a CT brain performed on the day of their clinic attendance (see Figs 1.1–1.3). Describe the abnormalities on each scan.

Figure 1.1 (Case 1.A) shows a hyperdense area in the right basal ganglia with mild perifocal oedema. The findings are in keeping with a subacute primary intracranial haemorrhage secondary to hypertension.

Figure 1.2 shows CT images before (Fig. 1.2(a)) and after (Fig. 1.2(b)) contrast administration. There is a solitary mass within the right frontal lobe with associated vasogenic oedema, which leads to effacement of the sulci and some compression of the right lateral ventricle. The lesion itself has a central necrotic core with irregular peripheral enhancement (arrow in Figure 1.6). These appearances are very suggestive of a high-grade glioma (e.g. a glioblastoma). The patient underwent resection of the tumour, and unfortunately the neuropathological findings confirmed this diagnosis.

Figure 1.3 (case C) shows a wedge-shaped area of low density in the inferolateral aspect of the left frontal lobe. The appearance is suggestive of an infarct in the left middle cerebral artery (MCA) territory.

5. The follow-up scans of Cases 1.A and 1.C are shown in Figs 1.4 and 1.5. What do you think is the most likely diagnosis now?

Figure 1.4 (Case 1.A 2 months later) shows a large hyperdense lesion with a central area of low density located in the right basal ganglia. There is also marked mass effect with midline shift. The appearances suggest haemorrhage into a tumour. Haemorrhage usually occurs in high-grade tumours, and in this case the patient was found to have a glioblastoma multiforme.

The patient in Case 1.C deteriorated with weight loss and worsening confusion over the subsequent months. Further brain imaging elsewhere showed a large mass in the left frontal lobe extending across the midline to the right frontal lobe. The underlying diagnosis was revised to a primary brain neoplasm, with glioblastoma multiforme the most likely type. Figure 1.5 shows the CT scan 3 months after intervention. At this stage, the patient had had a craniotomy for biopsy and debulking of the tumour, and he had also undergone radiotherapy. The scan shows oedema in the left frontal lobe, which may be due both to remaining tumour, and to after-effects from radiotherapy.

6. How often do patients referred to a dedicated TIA clinic turn out not to have had a cerebrovascular event?

Even though brain tumours are gradually progressing structural lesions, they may occasionally present with sudden onset symptoms which may be transient.

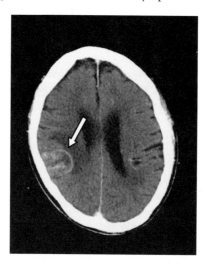

Fig. 1.6 CT brain from case 1.B shown again with an arrow indicating the lesion with a central necrotic core and irregular peripheral enhancement.

Table 1.2 Percentage of patients referred to dedicated 'TIA clinics' in whom a non-neurovascular diagnosis was made in the Oxford Vascular Study (OXVASC, 2002–2004) and the Oxford Community Stroke Project (OCSP, 1981–1986)

Diagnosis	OXVASC (%) (n = 112)	Diagnosis	OCSP (%) (n =317)
Migraine	22	Migraine	16
Anxiety	13	Syncope	15
Seizure	8	'Possible TIA'	15
Peripheral neuropathy	7	'Funny turn'	14
Arrhythmia	5	Isolated vertigo	10
Labyrinthine	5	Epilepsy	9
Postural hypotension	5	Transient global amnesia	5
Transient global amnesia	5	Lone bilateral blindness	4
Syncope	4	Isolated diplopia	1
Tumour or metastases	4	Drop attack	1
Cervical spine disease	3	Meningioma	1
Dementia	2	Miscellaneous	9
Myasthenia gravis	1		
Multiple sclerosis	1		
Parkinson's disease	1		
Miscellaneous	14		

One of the main reasons for brain imaging in patients with a suspected cerebrovascular event is to exclude other pathology. Studies have shown that approximately 3% of brain tumours are initially misdiagnosed as stroke. The majority of these (over 90%) are glioblastomas and meningiomas, while metastases account for 8% of cases. In addition to tumours, there is a large variety of other conditions that may mimic a cerebrovascular event at least in their initial presentation. Table 1.2 shows the diagnoses in patients who were referred to dedicated TIA clinics in Oxford with a suspected diagnosis of TIA or stroke, but who were found to have a non-vascular diagnosis. In general, approximately half of patients referred to a 'TIA-clinic' will turn out to have a different diagnosis than TIA or stroke.

Further discussion

In all three patients, the presentation was highly suggestive of a cerebrovascular event. Initial brain imaging did not clarify the diagnosis in two patients. These cases show that although brain tumours classically present with a slowly progressive history, this is not always the case, and occasionally they may mimic a stroke or TIA.

However, as two of the patients show, brain imaging, or at least CT imaging, is not always helpful. MRI is now more widely used in patients with cerebrovascular disease, which may increase the sensitivity for non-vascular lesions in patients with suspected cerebrovascular disease. However, sometimes it may only be progress over time that will clarify the diagnosis.

There are several mechanisms by which space-occupying lesions may cause sudden symptoms. They may cause focal seizures, which may cause a subsequent Todd's palsy, which may be diagnosed as an ischaemic event. As in Case 1.A, haemorrhage into a tumour can cause sudden-onset symptoms and it may not possible to determine whether a haemorrhage is caused by an underlying tumour (see Case 30). Therefore any patient with a haemorrhage in an unusual location should have further imaging, after resorption of the blood, to look for a potential causative lesion. Another mechanism by which a tumour may cause sudden-onset symptoms is through compression of an artery causing ischaemia, or potentially steal phenomena arising from a highly vascularized lesion.

Further reading

Amort M, Fluri F, Schäfer J, *et al.* (2011). Transient ischemic attack versus transient ischemic attack mimics: frequency, clinical characteristics and outcome. *Cerebrovasc Dis.*; **32**(1): 57–64.

Easton JD, Saver JL, Albers DW, *et al.* (2009). Definition and evaluation of transient ischemic attack a scientific statement for healthcare professionals from the American Heart Association/American Stroke Association Stroke Council. *Stroke*; **40**: 2276–93.

Hand PJ, Kwan J, Lindley RI, Dennis MS, Wardlaw JM. (2006). Distinguishing between stroke and mimic at the bedside: the brain attack study. *Stroke*; **37**(3): 769–75.

Koudstaal PJ, Gerritsma JG, van Gijn J. (1989). Clinical disagreement on the diagnosis of transient ischemic attack: is the patient or the doctor to blame? *Stroke*; **20**(2): 300–1.

Kraaijeveld CL, van Gijn J, Schouten HJ, Staal A. (1984). Interobserver agreement for the diagnosis of transient ischemic attacks. *Stroke*; **15**(4): 723–5.

Case 2

An 80-year-old retired engineer attended clinic with his wife. She reported that 2 days earlier, he had become suddenly confused with poor memory, asking the same question repeatedly and appearing disorientated. He complained of headache and was unable to perform his usual activities. These symptoms persisted for approximately 2 hours. He was then tired and a bit 'muddled'. He had no recollection of the event itself, but was otherwise back to normal. Neurological examination in clinic was entirely normal except that his Abbreviated Mental Test score was 7/10.

Questions

1. Give a list of causes of transient memory loss.
2. What does the CT brain (Fig. 2.1) show?
3. Review the subsequent MRI scans (Fig. 2.2). What is the most likely diagnosis based on these?
4. What are the advantages and disadvantages of CT and MRI in evaluating suspected cerebrovascular events? Comment on the MR sequences used in stroke, and the information that each provides.

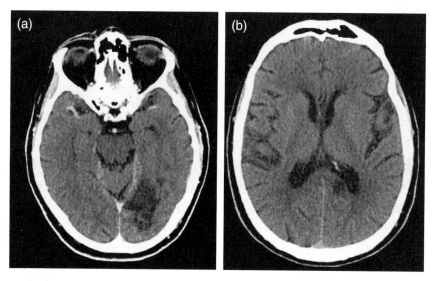

Fig. 2.1 CT head.

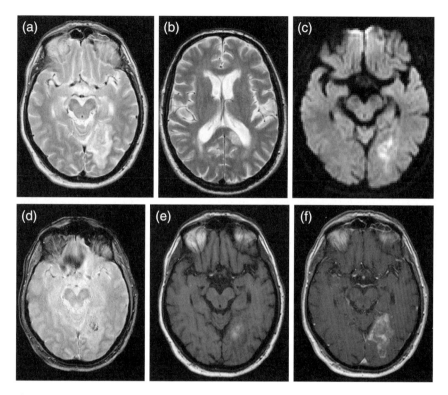

Fig. 2.2 MRI brain. Axial T2-weighted images (a, b), DWI (c), GRE (d) and axial contrast-enhanced T1-weighted images (e, f).

Answers

1. Give a list of causes of transient memory loss.

The patient presented with transient anterograde memory loss, i.e. an inability to retain new information. The repeated questioning, the symptom duration, and the quick return to normal, other than amnesia for the episode itself, would all be in keeping with transient global amnesia (TGA). This is a well-defined clinical entity, although the aetiology remains poorly understood. This condition appears to be entirely benign, even though it can cause considerable anxiety to the patient and especially to those witnessing an attack (see also Case 18).

The differential diagnosis for TGA includes:
- transient ischaemic amnesia
- transient migrainous amnesia
- transient epileptic amnesia
- transient psychogenic amnesia.

Often a more detailed history may help in making the diagnosis. For example, migraine and epilepsy will often cause recurrent events, whereas the risk of recurrence in TGA is generally low. Brain imaging may reveal ischaemic lesions, perhaps making a diagnosis of transient ischaemic amnesia more likely. In the current patient, the inability to continue with his usual activities would be unusual for TGA. Furthermore, the persisting cognitive deficit is not in keeping with this diagnosis. This may be due to a previously unrecognized dementia, but is a cause for concern and warrants further investigation.

2. What does the CT head (Fig. 2.1) show?

The CT brain scan shows a hypodense lesion in the left occipital lobe with mild contrast enhancement. There is a second lesion within the splenium of the corpus callosum on the left (see arrows in Fig. 2.3).

While subacute infarction was considered, the lesion distribution was thought to be unusual for a vascular aetiology, and the most likely diagnosis was felt to be a tumour in the left occipital lobe, with a satellite lesion in the splenium of the corpus callosum. Further assessment with MRI was recommended.

3. Review the subsequent MRI scans (Fig. 2.2). What is the most likely diagnosis based on these?

The MRI scans confirmed the presence of lesions in the medial occipital lobe (Fig. 2.4(a)) and the left posterior corpus callosum (Fig. 2.4(b)). The lesions have slightly restricted diffusion on diffusion-weighted imaging (DWI) (Fig. 2.4(c)). Gradient echo imaging (GRE) shows some haemorrhagic transformation within the lesion (Fig. 2.4(d)). On T1-weighted imaging, the lesion is partially hyperdense (Fig. 2.4(e)), suggesting haemorrhagic transformation. There is now avid contrast enhancement (Fig. 2.4(f), T1 + gadolinium), consistent with breakdown of the

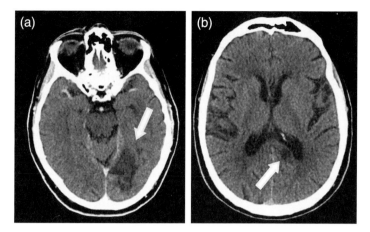

Fig. 2.3 CT brain indicating lesions in left occipital lobe (a) and splenium of the corpus callosum (b).

blood–brain barrier. While a neoplasm cannot be entirely excluded, the lesion appearance, in particular the restricted diffusion, the presence of haemorrhagic transformation, and the fact that both lesions are located in the territory of the left posterior cerebral artery make a diagnosis of infarction much more likely.

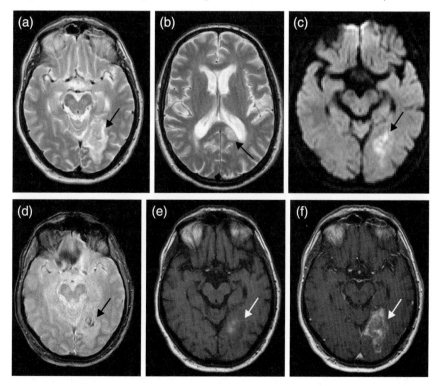

Fig. 2.4 MRI brain indicating lesions in left occipital lobe and splenium of the corpus callosum.

To resolve any remaining uncertainty as to whether the diagnosis was an infarct or a tumour, a follow-up MRI scan was done 6 weeks later (Fig. 2.5). The size of the lesion had decreased on the T2-weighted imaging (Fig. 2.5(a)), there was no longer any evidence of restricted diffusion (Fig. 2.5(b)), and contrast enhancement was much less marked (Fig. 2.5(c)). A diagnosis of left posterior cerebral artery infarction was confirmed.

4. What are the advantages and disadvantages of CT and MRI in evaluating suspected cerebrovascular events? Comment on the MR sequences used in stroke, and the information that each provides.

CT brain scanning is still the most commonly used imaging modality in patients with suspected stroke or TIA. The advantages of CT scanning are that it is widely available, it can be done very quickly, and it is sensitive in diagnosing acute haemorrhage. Disadvantages of CT are that hyperacute infarction may be difficult to diagnose by inexperienced observers, imaging of the posterior fossa is difficult because of artefacts, there is a relatively high dose of radiation, particularly when more advanced CT techniques are used, and it is less sensitive than MRI in showing non-vascular lesions. Beyond the acute stage, CT cannot differentiate between haemorrhage and infarction, with small haemorrhages often resolving within days. Multimodal CT, including CT perfusion imaging and CT angiography (CTA), is now available. The use of CTA or MRA depends strongly on local preference, and the amount of information these techniques provide is probably similar. However, processing time and radiation dose are higher for CTA. CT perfusion imaging may be helpful in determining which acute stroke patients might benefit from thrombolysis, but it is not yet widely used.

The main disadvantages of MRI scanning are that it is less widely available than CT, it is more prone to movement artefact than CT, and the duration of a scan is longer. All of this makes it difficult to scan acutely ill patients. However, with ongoing development of MRI and the availability of stronger magnets, scan times have reduced, which makes MRI scanning feasible even in less cooperative patients.

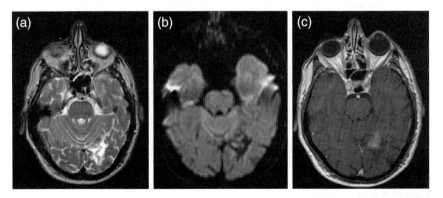

Fig. 2.5 Follow-up MRI: T2-weighted axial image (a), DWI (b), and T1-weighted image with contrast (c).

A further disadvantage of MRI is that it cannot be used in some patients (e.g. patients with cardiac pacemakers or metal implants). These contraindications may be difficult to elicit if the patient is unwell, confused, or dysphasic. Other patients find scans difficult to tolerate because they are claustrophobic.

MRI has several advantages over CT. These are particularly obvious in patients with TIA or minor stroke, in whom CT will often be normal. MRI sequences frequently used in patients with suspected cerebrovascular disease are as follows.

♦ *Structural imaging* with T2-weighted sequences, FLAIR (fluid attenuated inversion recovery), which gives images similar to standard T2-weighted imaging, but with suppression of the high signal from cerebrospinal fluid (CSF), or, less commonly, T1-weighted sequences without and with contrast. These sequences predominantly aim to obtain anatomical information and look for the presence of structural lesions of any aetiology. T1-weighted sequences are often used to assess whether a lesion exhibits contrast enhancement, i.e if there is evidence of blood-brain-barrier-breakdown. This may occur in inflammatory lesions and tumours. It is important to note that it also occurs in ischaemic stroke, which may sometimes lead to confusion and to a misdiagnosis of an infarct as a tumour.

♦ *Diffusion-weighted imaging (DWI):* DWI looks for the presence of cytotoxic oedema, which occurs in acute ischaemia. Acute ischaemic lesions will appear as bright white. The high signal will resolve over some weeks, and this sequence is particularly useful for diagnosing acute infarction and for differentiating acute from chronic ischaemic lesions in patients with previous cerebrovascular events. Sometimes on DWI, chronic lesions may still have high signal caused by 'T2 shine through'. In such cases, the apparent diffusion coefficient (ADC) map is helpful. The ADC will be low, showing as low signal on the ADC map, for up to 2 weeks after infarction and will then increase. Therefore recent infarction will appear as high signal on DWI and low signal on ADC (Fig. 2.6) It is also

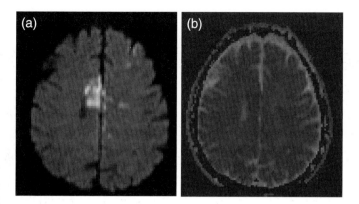

Fig. 2.6 (a) The DWI shows high signal in the right anterior cerebral artery territory, suggestive of acute infarction. (b) The low signal in the same region on the ADC map confirms that the infarct is acute.

important to bear in mind that high signal on DWI is not entirely specific for infarction. Cytotoxic oedema may also occur in inflammatory lesions, cerebral abscesses, and some high-grade tumours.

◆ *GRE* or *Susceptibility weighted imaging (SWI):* GRE or SWI are particularly sensitive to haemorrhage, which will show as low signal. These sequences are helpful in differentiating haemorrhage from infarction, and they may also show 'microhaemorrhages', which may occur in hypertension or amyloid angiopathy. In contrast with CT, which cannot differentiate between haemorrhage and infarct beyond the acute stage, chronic haemorrhage is still visible on MRI and can be differentiated from ischaemic lesions.

◆ *MR angiography (MRA):* This can be done as time-of-flight MRA (TOF-MRA), which does not require contrast, or as contrast-enhanced MRA (CE-MRA), which requires the use of gadolinium but provides higher-quality images. As opposed to Doppler ultrasound, which, at least in the UK, is mainly used to assess the extracranial carotid arteries, MRA can be used to study the vessels of both the anterior and posterior circulation, and it also provides images of the intracranial circulation. Therefore it provides much more detailed information on the location and extent of atheromatous disease or vascular lesions of other aetiology (e.g. arterial dissections or vasculitis).

Further reading

Muir KW, Buchan A, von Kummer R, Rother J (2006). Imaging of acute stroke. *Lancet Neurol*; **5**: 755–68.

Owen D, Paranandi B, Sivakumar R, Seevaratnam M (2007). Classical diseases revisited: transient global amnesia. *Postgrad Med J*; **83**: 236–9.

Case 3

Case 3.A

A 49-year-old man awoke in the morning with vertigo. He was very unsteady on walking, always veering to the left. He had developed hiccups and vomited on a few occasions. He spilt some hot water over his legs trying to make himself a cup of tea, but did not perceive the water as hot on his right leg. The patient had a history of hypertension, he was a smoker, and he had had a stroke with right-sided sensory loss 2 years before. On examination there was a left Horner's syndrome, reduced perception of pinprick and temperature on the left side of the face and the right side of the body, coarse gaze-evoked nystagmus to the left, and a left-sided ataxia.

Case 3.B

A 74-year-old hypertensive man with a long history of chronic dizziness became aware of a sudden worsening of the dizziness while walking around in his flat. He also noticed bright sparkling colourful stars in his right visual hemifield and repeatedly bumped into objects on his right. Clinical examination showed a right hemianopia, and MRI brain confirmed the clinical diagnosis of a left occipital infarct.

Questions

1. Which part of the brain is affected in Case 3.A? What do you call this syndrome? Which artery is usually involved?
2. List the typical symptoms and signs of this syndrome and name the affected structures.
3. The MRA and DWI of patient A is shown in Fig. 3.1. Describe your findings.
4. How would you treat these patients?

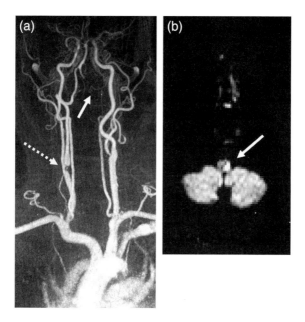

Fig. 3.1 Contrast-enhanced MRA (a) and DWI (b) for Case 3.A.

Answers

1. Which part of the brain is affected in Case 3.A? What do you call this syndrome? Which artery is usually involved?

This patient presents with a lateral medullary syndrome. This is often also called 'Wallenberg syndrome' after Adolf Wallenberg (1862–1949), a German neurologist, who first described this syndrome in 1895. As the name suggests, the syndrome is caused by an infarct affecting the dorsolateral medulla. It is caused by occlusion of the posterior inferior cerebellar artery, although vascular imaging will often show an occlusion of the vertebral artery.

2. List the typical symptoms and signs of this syndrome and name the affected structures.

The typical symptoms and signs of the lateral medullary syndrome and the affected brainstem structures are listed in Table 3.1.

3. The MRA and DWI of patient A is shown in Fig. 3.1. Describe your findings.

The MR angiogram (MRA) for Case 3.A (Fig. 3.1(a)) shows an occlusion of the left vertebral artery (short arrow). Compared with the right, the V3 segment and the proximal V4 segment of the left vertebral artery are not visible. There is retrograde filling of the distal V4 segment of the left vertebral artery from the basilar artery. The MRA also shows a right carotid stenosis at the bifurcation (dashed arrow). The diffusion-weighted image (Fig. 3.1(b)) shows the left lateral medullary infarct.

Table 3.1 Symptoms and signs of lateral medullary syndrome

Symptom/sign	Affected structure
Hiccups	Uncertain, but may be vagus nucleus or tractus solitarius
Dysphagia	Ipsilateral nucleus ambiguous (supplying CN IX and X) and tractus solitarius
Hoarse voice	Glossopharyngeal and vagus fibres
Ipsilateral	
Facial loss of pain and temperature sensation	Ipsilateral trigeminal tracts
Horner's syndrome	Descending sympathetic fibres
Ataxia	Inferior cerebellar peduncle
Nystagmus	Inferior cerebellar peduncle
Contralateral	
Loss of pain and temperature perception of limbs and body	Spinothalamic tract

The MRA for Case 3.B (Fig. 3.2) shows a hypoplastic right vertebral artery, which ends in the right posterior inferior cerebellar artery and does not contribute to flow in the basilar artery (short white arrow). There is a short tight stenosis in the V4-segment of the left vertebral artery (thin white dashed arrow). There is also a stenosis in the petrous segment of the right internal carotid artery (ICA) (thin long solid arrow) and of the left ICA in the siphon (thick dotted arrow). In this patient, both anterior cerebral arteries are filled from the right ICA.

4. How would you treat these patients?

Both patients have had relatively minor symptoms. They may require some rehabilitation, but treatment will mainly be directed at secondary stroke prevention. Certainly, the risk of recurrence after a posterior circulation ischaemic event is high, up to 15–20% in the first month. The risk is three times higher in patients with a vertebral or basilar artery stenosis of at least 50% than in patients without stenotic disease (90-day risk of 46% vs. 21% in a population-based study (Marquardt *et al.* 2009)). In contrast to endarterectomy in symptomatic carotid stenosis, there is no established surgical option for vertebral artery stenosis, although angioplasty and stenting have recently become available. However, virtually no randomized data of the risks versus the benefits of this intervention exist. Case series give a peri-procedural risk of stroke of 2–3% in the proximal vertebral artery, and of up to 10% in the distal (intracranial)

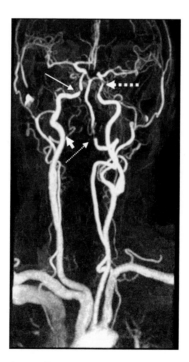

Fig. 3.2 Contrast-enhanced MRA for Case 3.B.

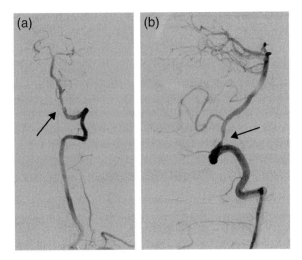

Fig. 3.3 Intra-arterial angiogram prior to stenting of the left vertebral artery stenosis. The arrows indicate the stenosis in (a) the anteroposterior (AP) view and (b) the lateral view.

vertebral artery. Two randomized trials of angioplasty/stenting versus best medical treatment alone in patients with recently symptomatic vertebral artery stenosis are ongoing. The patient in Case 3.B, who had a well-circumscribed vertebral artery stenosis, was included in one of the trials and was randomized to intervention. The distal

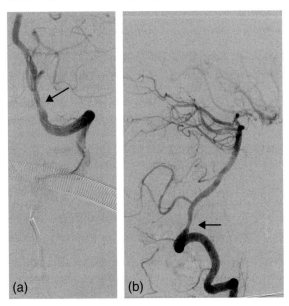

Fig. 3.4 Angiogram after angioplasty of the left vertebral artery stenosis. The arrows indicate that there is a mild residual stenosis, but that this is much improved compared with the pre-stenting images in Fig. 3.3.

vertebral artery stenosis was angioplastied with a good result (see Figs 3.3 and 3.4) and no immediate complications. The patient continues on his secondary prevention medication. Ideally, any patients with vertebral artery stenosis should be treated within such a trial.

The patient in Case 3.A had a vertebral artery occlusion. In the anterior circulation the risk of further events distal to an occluded vessel is lower than distal to a stenosis, and generally patients are treated with medication alone. This is also the approach in the posterior circulation, and this patient was managed conservatively. Medical management consists of giving antiplatelet agents, cholesterol-lowering drugs, and careful control of blood pressure. In the past, anticoagulation was used in posterior circulation disease after initial reports of symptom improvement in patients with vertebrobasilar ischaemia. However, more recently, the WASID study found no overall benefit of anticoagulation over aspirin in patients with intracranial atheroma, including patients with intracranial posterior circulation disease. Its use is now not generally recommended, and patients should receive antiplatelet drugs. In patients with vessel occlusion or bilateral severe stenosis, it is advisable not to lower blood pressure too much to ensure that an adequate perfusion pressure is maintained. We generally aim to keep the blood pressure slightly above 'normal' at around 130/85mmHg, although this will have to be individually tailored to each patient and their symptoms and usual blood pressure.

Further reading

Chimowitz MI, Lynn MJ, Howlett-Smith H, *et al.* for the Warfarin–Aspirin Symptomatic Intracranial Disease Trial Investigators (2005). Comparison of warfarin and aspirin for symptomatic intracranial arterial stenosis. *N Engl J Med*; **352**: 1305–16.

Compter A, van der Worp HB, Schonewille WJ, *et al.* (2008). VAST: Vertebral Artery Stenting Trial. Protocol for a randomised safety and feasibility trial. *Trials*; **9**: 65.

Gulli G, Khan S, Markus HS (2009). Vertebrobasilar stenosis predicts high early recurrent stroke risk in posterior circulation stroke and TIA. *Stroke*; **40**: 2732–7.

Marquardt L, Kuker W, Chandratheva A, Geraghty O, Rothwell PM (2009). Incidence and prognosis of ≥50% symptomatic vertebral or basilar artery stenosis: prospective population-based study. *Brain*; **132**: 982–8.

Savitz SJ, Caplan LR (2005). Current concepts: Vertebrobasilar disease. *N Engl J Med*; **352**: 2618–26.

Vertebral Artery Ischaemia Stenting Trial (VIST). Available online at www.vist.sgul.ac.uk. Accessed 7 November 2011.

Case 4

A 74-year-old woman presented to the medical take with confusion that appeared to have come on gradually over a few days. There was a past history of hypertension and she was taking bendroflumethiazide. She had otherwise been fit and well. On examination, she was drowsy and unable to answer questions or follow commands. Her cheeks appeared flushed. She was apyrexial with an irregular pulse of 100bpm and blood pressure of 110/70mmHg. There were no splinter haemorrhages. Examination of the cardiovascular system showed a grossly displaced apex, loud pansystolic murmur, low-pitched diastolic murmur, and a loud first heart sound. The jugular venous pressure (JVP) was raised 6cm with evidence of systolic (CV) waves, and there was mild ankle swelling. Cranial nerves (CN) appeared intact, fundi were normal, and examination of the limbs showed increased tone on the right and an extensor right plantar response. There was multifocal myoclonus.

The patient was commenced on intravenous aciclovir pending brain imaging results. Blood tests, including full blood count (FBC), liver function tests (LFTs), calcium (Ca), and glucose were unremarkable except for a C-reactive protein (CRP) of 37mg/L and a creatinine (Cr) of 166μmol/L. The chest X-ray (CXR) and electrocardiogram (ECG) are shown in Figs 4.1 and 4.2.

Questions

1. What do the examination findings, CXR (Fig 4.1.), and ECG (Fig 4.2.) suggest?
2. Given the answer to question 1 and the other investigation results, what is the most likely cause of the neurological findings?
3. How would you confirm your diagnosis?
4. How would you manage this patient?

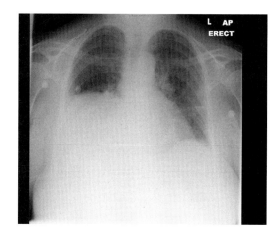

Fig. 4.1 CXR.

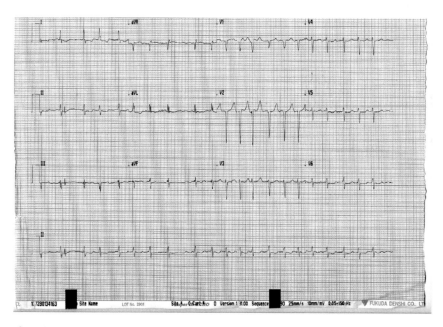

Fig. 4.2 ECG.

Answers

1. What do the examination findings, CXR (Fig 4.1.), and ECG (Fig 4.2.) suggest?

The cardiac findings suggest atrial fibrillation (AF) in association with mixed mitral valve disease and tricuspid regurgitation.

The ECG confirms AF. The CXR shows cardiomegaly with an enlarged left atrium and a pleural effusion. On clinical examination, there is AF and elevation of the venous pressure with CV waves caused by tricuspid regurgitation. The apex is displaced, consistent with cardiomegaly, and there is a loud pansystolic murmur at the apex indicating mitral (and tricuspid) regurgitation. The loud S1 and mid-diastolic murmur indicate mitral stenosis. Thus the patient has mixed mitral valve disease with secondary right heart changes, probably due to rheumatic fever.

2. Given the answer to question 1 and the other investigation results, what is the most likely cause of the neurological findings?

The most likely diagnosis is multiple cerebral embolism secondary to AF in the context of mitral valve disease.

Although this patient's presentation with confusion and myoclonus is atypical for stroke, this remains the most likely diagnosis in view of her underlying cardiac disease which was previously unknown and therefore not treated (see Case 37, Table 37.1). AF is a strong risk factor for stroke, and the risk rises further if there is associated rheumatic heart disease (see Cases 22 and 37 for further discussion).

Myoclonus has been reported in association with brainstem stroke but is not widely recognized in association with infarcts not affecting the brainstem. The differential diagnosis includes the following:

- Encephalopathy
  - metabolic derangement
  - hypoxic brain damage (e.g. after cardiac arrest)
  - drug toxicity
  - Wernicke's encepahlopathy
  - Hashimoto's encephalopathy
- Central nervous system (CNS) infection
  - herpes simplex encephalitis
  - sporadic Creutzfeld–Jakob disease (CJD)
- Vascular
  - cerebral venous sinus thrombosis (CVST)
  - vasculitis
- Non-convulsive status epilepticus

In this case, common metabolic abnormalities were excluded, and there was no reason to suspect drug toxicity or alcohol-related problems. Hashimoto's encephalopathy causes confusion, and may be associated with stroke-like episodes, seizures, myoclonus and fluctuation in mental state. Brain imaging is usually normal. Herpes simplex encephalitis should always be considered in patients presenting with confusion or altered behaviour, particularly if there is a fever or prodromal illness. CVST may present with confusion and reduced level of consciousness (see Cases 5 and 17). There is usually a history of headache, and fundoscopy often shows papilloedema. There were no risk factors for CVST in this patient. CNS vasculitis (see Cases 11, 15, and 25) usually causes confusion or change in level of consciousness associated with focal neurological signs. Space-occupying lesions are a common cause of altered behaviour, although one would not usually expect multifocal myoclonus. Non-convulsive status epilepticus causes altered behaviour and impaired alertness. Seizures occurring *de novo* in older people are most commonly caused by cerebrovascular disease which may have been previously undiagnosed.

3. How would you confirm your diagnosis?

Brain imaging and echocardiography are required to confirm the diagnosis.

A CT brain scan would usually be performed first in cases such as this to identify the presence of any ischaemic, inflammatory, or neoplastic lesions, and to exclude or confirm the presence of haemorrhage. In this patient, the CT showed evidence of multiple ischaemic strokes. The subsequent MRI/DWI brain was done to determine the age of the lesions more accurately. It confirmed the presence of multiple acute lesions affecting both cerebral hemispheres consistent with an embolic source (Fig. 4.3), although such findings may also be seen in cerebral vasculitis (see Cases 11 and 25) and intravascular large B-cell lymphoma (IVBCL) (see Case 50). DWI is of particular use in distinguishing acute from chronic infarction and thus in determining the aetiology of the stroke (see Case 32). The cause of any stroke should always be established where possible since this has implications for secondary prevention.

Echocardiogram confirmed mitral valve disease with stenosis being predominant (estimated valve area of $1.1cm^2$). There was marked tricuspid regurgitation in the context of severe secondary pulmonary hypertension (estimated pulmonary artery (PA) pressure of 55mmHg). Left and right ventricular function was normal. A subsequent transoesophageal echocardiogram showed an atrial septal defect (ASD) with reversed right–left flow.

4. How would you manage this patient?

Management includes acute stroke unit transfer and cardiology work-up, and eventually anticoagulation.

The patient should be transferred to the acute stroke unit for optimal care, including prevention of post-stroke complications, and early rehabilitation. Anticoagulation is required to prevent further embolic events, assuming that there are no contraindications. There are no data to guide decisions about when to start anticoagulation. Current UK guidelines recommend immediate aspirin followed

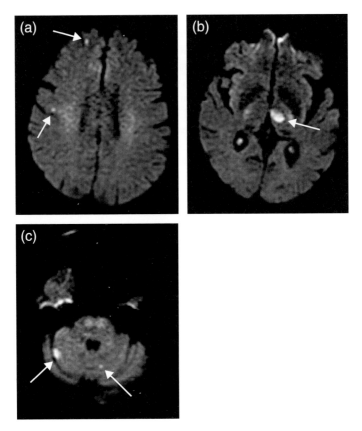

Fig. 4.3 Diffusion-weighted MRI brain. This shows multiple acute ischaemic infarcts in the right hemisphere (a), left thalamus (b), and both cerebellar hemispheres (c). Multiple infarcts in multiple vascular territories strongly suggest a cardioembolic aetiology.

by introduction of anticoagulation after 2 weeks since there is a risk of precipitating haemorrhagic transformation. Cardiology input is required to guide management of the patient's mitral valve disease.

The patient's myoclonus resolved after about 48 hours and her level of consciousness returned to normal on the stroke unit. She made a good neurological recovery although there was some residual unsteadiness and memory difficulty (see Case 8 for review of post-stroke cognitive impairment). The patient was seen by the cardiologists as an outpatient. They did not feel that intervention was justified at this stage, but stated that palliative mitral valve balloon angioplasty was a possible option if she were to become breathless. They also did not propose intervention for the ASD. Given the flow reversal, this may have been a possible contributing factor to this patient's infarcts by allowing paradoxical emboli. However, it is uncertain if the risk of further events would have been reduced by any procedure. While ASDs are relatively rare, paradoxical embolism through a patent foramen ovale (PFO) and its management is a more commonly debated topic in patients with otherwise cryptogenic stroke. This issue is discussed further in Case 48.

Further reading

Babarro EG, Rego AR, González-Juanatey JR (2009). Cardioembolic stroke: call for a multidisciplinary approach. *Cerebrovasc Dis*; **27** (Suppl 1): 82–7.

Medi C, Hankey GJ, Freedman SB (2010). Stroke risk and antithrombotic strategies in atrial fibrillation. *Stroke*; **41**: 2705–13.

http://www.nice.org.uk/nicemedia/pdf/CG036niceguideline.pdf.

http://www.rcplondon.ac.uk/pubs/books/stroke/stroke_guidelines_2ed.pdf.

http://www.sign.ac.uk/guidelines/fulltext/108/index.html.

Case 5

A 15-year-old girl of Pakistani origin presented with a 10-day history of worsening left-sided headache and vomiting. She was admitted to her local hospital after a generalized seizure. Apart from mild asthma and acne there was no past medical history of note. She had been started on minocycline for her acne 2 months earlier. She had three younger sisters, who were all well. Her parents were first cousins. Clinical examination on admission was normal. In particular, she was not overweight and there was no papilloedema. Her non-contrast CT scan is shown in Fig. 5.1.

The patient deteriorated the next day and became increasingly drowsy. A cerebral angiogram was done. The images are shown in Figs 5.2(a) and 5.2(b).

Questions

1. Describe the findings in Fig. 5.1. What is the diagnosis?
2. Describe the findings in Figs 5.2 and 5.3. Do you see any association between the appearances in these figures? If so, what?
3. What investigations would you perform to confirm the diagnosis?
4. How would you treat this patient?
5. What is the relevance of this condition and its treatment in stroke due to atheromatous disease?

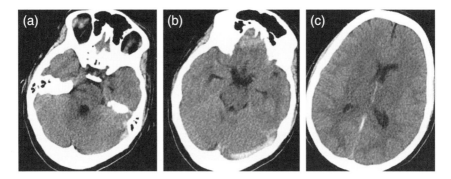

Fig. 5.1 Non-contrast CT brain.

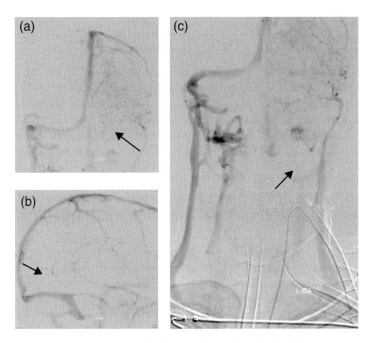

Fig. 5.2 Cerebral venogram, AP projections (a, c), and lateral view (b).

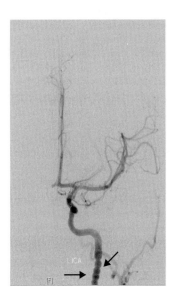

Fig. 5.3 Cerebral intra-arterial angiogram (AP view), left ICA injection.

Answers

1. Describe the findings in Fig. 5.1. What is the diagnosis?

Figure 5.1 is an unenhanced CT scan, which shows high signal in the left sigmoid sinus (Fig. 5.1(a)), the transverse sinus (Fig. 5.1 (b)), and the straight sinus (Fig. 5.1(c)). The likely diagnosis is CVST. It is important to note that this is an *un*enhanced CT scan, so the high signal in the sinuses is due to thrombus. In a contrast enhanced CT, the high signal would represent contrast medium and thrombus would show up as a filling defect with a lower signal than the surrounding contrast-filled vessels (see also Case 17).

2. Describe the findings in Figs 5.2 and 5.3. Do you see any association between the appearances in these figures? If so, what?

Figure 5.2 shows lack of filling of the left transverse (a), straight (b), and sigmoid sinus and the left internal jugular vein (c), consistent with a diagnosis of venous sinus thrombosis. Figure 5.3 shows changes in the left ICA. The artery shows a string and bead appearance, which is consistent with fibromuscular dysplasia (FMD). The association of venous sinus thrombosis and FMD has been described in homocystinuria.

Homocystinuria is a genetic disorder, which is usually autosomal recessive and is characterized by abnormalities in homocysteine metabolism. Homocysteine is metabolized by either the re-methylation pathway, which requires vitamin B_{12} and folate as cofactors, or the trans-sulphuration pathway, which requires pyridoxine as a cofactor. The enzymes that are involved are methionine synthase, methylene tetrahydrofolate reductase (MTHFR) and cystathionine β-synthase (CBS), respectively. Defects in these pathways, of which CBS deficiency is the most common, lead to an accumulation of homocysteine in the blood and urine. Classically, patients present with a marfanoid stature, downward dislocation of the lens, and thromboembolic events at a young age, with half of all patients estimated to have had a vascular event by the age of 30 years. However, more recent studies have suggested that many defect carriers will not necessarily develop the full phenotype and remain unrecognized, with perhaps the only manifestation of the disease being premature ischaemic events. Treatment of homocystinuria is directed at reducing homocysteine levels. This can be achieved by reducing its production by having a diet low in methionine, which is the amino acid that is transformed into homocysteine. Homocysteine levels can also be reduced by increasing its metabolism. To achieve this, patients are given high doses of pyridoxine and, if not sufficient, of vitamin B_{12} and folate. Furthermore, supplementation with betaine can also lower homocysteine levels. Finally, patients may require supplementation with cysteine, which may only be formed in insufficient amounts if there is CBS deficiency. Treatment efficacy is monitored by measuring homocysteine levels.

3. What investigations would you perform to confirm the diagnosis?

To diagnose homocystinuria, urine is screened for sulphur-containing amino acids. If positive, methionine, homocysteine, and cystathionine levels should be determined. Blood levels of homocysteine and methionine can also be measured. Cystathionine synthase activity can be determined from cultured fibroblasts. Genetic testing is available, though more widely used for prenatal testing or to test for asymptomatic carriers. In this patient, investigations confirmed the suspected diagnosis of homocystinuria due to CBS deficiency.

4. How would you treat this patient?

There are two treatment issues in this patient: treatment of the CVST, and treatment of the underlying homocystinuria. A third aspect is treatment of her currently asymptomatic arterial FMD (see also Case 36).

Treatment of CVST is described in more detail in Case 17. In the current patient, prognosis without intervention appeared poor because she had a reduced level of consciousness and she continued to deteriorate despite anticoagulation having been started after the initial imaging. Therefore the decision was made to proceed to local thrombolysis. The straight sinus was recanalized successfully, and the patient awoke the next day without any focal deficit. She was anticoagulated for 6 months, and then started on aspirin which was used to prevent complications from her dysplastic arteries. Treatment with high-dose pyridoxine, vitamin B_{12}, and folate led to a significant drop in her homocysteine levels.

5. What is the relevance of this condition and its treatment in stroke due to atheromatous disease?

In recent years, studies have suggested that high homocysteine levels are a risk factor for ischaemic stroke due to atheromatous disease, even if they are lower than the levels found in homocystinuria. It is still unclear how homocysteine increases the risk for atheroma, but it is thought to promote proliferation of vascular smooth muscle cells, to induce endothelial dysfunction, and to facilitate oxidative arterial injury. It may also alter the coagulant properties of blood, thus promoting thrombosis. Homocysteine levels depend on a number of environmental factors. For example, they can be increased by smoking, renal disease, hypothyroidism, and older age. Enzyme defects in the metabolic pathways for homocysteine and nutritional deficiencies, namely of folate, vitamin B_{12}, and pyridoxine, may also contribute. Given that these three vitamins are essential for homocysteine metabolism, there have now been a number of studies looking at whether vitamin supplementation will decrease the risk of stroke. The largest of these studies (VITATOPS) showed that the risk of ischaemic stroke was not reduced significantly in patients receiving supplementation with folate, vitamin B_{12}, and pyridoxine compared with patients who received placebo. In addition, other studies suggested that the high homocysteine levels found in patients with stroke may follow vascular events rather than contribute to their risk. Indeed, some prospective studies failed to confirm the association between homocysteine and atheromatous disease, which had previously been described predominantly in cross-sectional studies. Overall, although many studies have shown an association between increased homocysteine levels and atheromatous disease, the mechanism of this association and the role of reducing homocysteine levels in preventing vascular events still remain uncertain and require further research. However, it appears worthwhile to check homocysteine levels in patients with premature atheromatous disease to detect more severe underlying metabolic defects and to identify any potentially treatable factors that may be contributing to a patient's risk of having ischaemic events.

Further reading

Chauveheid MP, Lidove O, Papo T (2008). Adult-onset homocystinuria arteriopathy mimics fibromuscular dysplasia. *Am J Med*; **121**: e5–6

Hankey GJ, Eikelboom JW (2001). Homocysteine and stroke. *Curr Opin Neurol*; **14**: 95–102.

VITATOPS Trial Study Group (2010). B vitamins in patients with recent transient ischaemic attack or stroke in the VITAmins TO Prevent Stroke (VITATOPS) trial: a randomised, double-blind, parallel, placebo-controlled trial. *Lancet Neurol*; **9**: 855–65.

Case 6

Case 6.A

A 74-year-old man was referred to the TIA clinic by his GP. One week previously, he had developed sudden-onset difficulty in using his right arm and leg whilst gardening. On direct questioning, he described a mild weakness of the right limbs that had gradually resolved over a few days. He had no past medical history and was normally fit and active, and his hobbies included playing bridge competitively.

On examination, his blood pressure was 175/80mmHg, there was mild inattention to the right, and he had bilateral extensor plantar reflexes. He was diagnosed with a left parietal stroke and was prescribed aspirin, a statin, and antihypertensive medication. Carotid Dopplers were normal.

Case 6.B

An 80-year-old man presented to the TIA clinic with a brief episode of horizontal double vision which came on whilst he was watching television. The abnormality lasted for 10 minutes before resolving completely. He called the out-of-hours GP who found no abnormality. He had a past history of several strokes.

- 1995: vertigo, ataxia, left visual field defect, left arm and leg weakness.
- May 2005: dizziness and ataxia, left visual field defect. A CT showed an old right occipital infarct and multiple old small infarcts in both hemispheres.
- November 2005: episode of transient left sided weakness. MRI/MRA showed an old right PCA infarct involving the medial temporal lobe, right lower occipital lobe, and a smaller left cerebellar infarct, and a lacunar infarct in the right lentiform nucleus. Haemosiderin deposition (microbleeds) were noted in the cerebellum, thalamus, and left parietal white matter.
- January 2006: further episode of ataxia. MRI showed a subacute haematoma in the left cerebellar hemisphere on a background of several infarcted areas, including the right inferior temporal and occipital regions.
- February 2006: further posterior circulation event.

Case 6.C

An 84-year-old man was referred to the geratology clinic with poor mobility, falls, and poor memory. He had previously been seen in the memory clinic and had been diagnosed with vascular cognitive impairment. There was a past history of hypertension. On examination, he was frail and in sinus rhythm with a significant postural blood pressure drop. He had a stooped posture and unsteady gait with shuffling steps. However, he had good upper limb mobility and there was no cogwheeling. MMSE was 23/30 and this was similar to his scores from the two previous years. He had a CT brain scan that was reported as showing small vessel disease. He was referred for physiotherapy and his antihypertensive medication was reduced. One year later, he presented as an emergency with a parietal lobar haemorrhage. He underwent a CT brain scan followed by MRI (Fig. 6.1).

Questions

1. Describe the abnormalities on the brain imaging in Fig. 6.1 and give a differential diagnosis for the MRI appearance.
2. What is the diagnosis that fits all three cases and what are the different clinical syndromes associated with this diagnosis?
3. What advice would you give regarding medication?

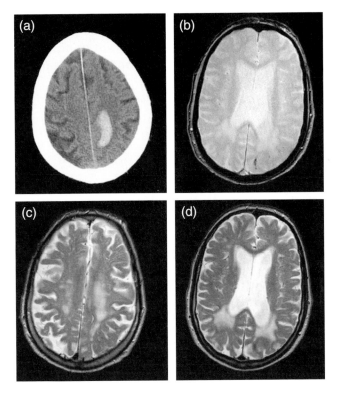

Fig. 6.1 CT brain (a) and MRI brain: GRE (b), and axial T2-weighted images (c, d).

Answers

1. Describe the abnormalities on the brain imaging in Fig. 6.1 and give a differential diagnosis for the MRI appearance

The images shown in Fig. 6.1 are shown again in Fig. 6.2 with arrows indicating the abnormalities. The CT brain slice in Fig. 6.2(a) shows a superficial posterior left parietal haemorrhage. The arrow in Fig. 6.2(b) is pointing to a left occipital microbleed shown on GRE. The T2-weighted images ((c) and (d)) show extensive bilateral hyperintense signal changes in both hemispheres.

The differential diagnosis of the radiological findings of widespread white matter changes and multiple microhaemorrhages is cerebral amyloid angiopathy (CAA), hypertensive small vessel disease, and CADASIL (see Case 28). In CAA, any larger haemorrhages are typically lobar, whereas in hypertensive small vessel disease,

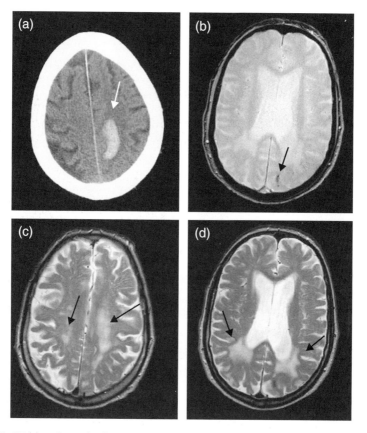

Fig. 6.2 CT (a) and MRI (b–d) showing left parietal haemorrhage (a), left occipital microbleed (b), and extensive white matter changes (c,d).

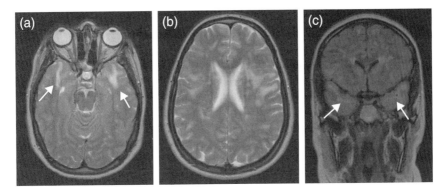

Fig. 6.3 (a, b) T2-weighted axial images and (c) coronal FLAIR of a patient with CADASIL. The images show widespread white matter changes, which also affect the anterior temporal lobes (arrows).

haemorrhages are usually located in the basal ganglia. In CADASIL, white matter changes are typically also found in the temporal lobes, whereas these are only rarely affected in CAA and hypertensive small vessel disease (Figs 6.3 and 6.4). The imaging appearances here are most in keeping with CAA.

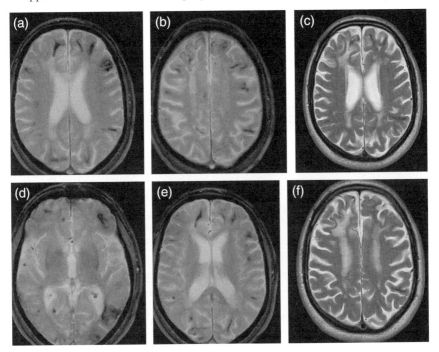

Fig. 6.4 GRE showing multiple areas of old haemorrhage including subcortical haemorrhages and microbleeds (a, b, d, e), and T2-weighted images (c, f) showing widespread white matter changes in a patient with CAA. The temporal lobe white matter changes which are seen in CADASIL are not present in CAA.

2. What is the diagnosis that fits all three cases and what are the different clinical syndromes associated with this diagnosis?

CAA is the diagnosis that fits all three cases. CAA (see Table 6.1 for diagnostic criteria) is associated with:

- recurrent lobar haemorrhage
- subcortical ischaemia
- migraine
- dementia
- cortical haemorrhage
- seizures.

The three cases outlined above together illustrate recurrent stroke including lobar haemorrhage, gait disorder, cognitive impairment, confluent white matter changes, and haematomas of different ages as clinical presenting features of CAA. Other relatively common causes of non-traumatic lobar haemorrhage include:

- lobar extension of a putaminal haemorrhage
- haemorrhagic transformation of an ischaemic stroke
- arteriovenous malformation (AVM)
- haemorrhagic tumour (see Case 30).

Differentiation of CAA from these conditions depends on the clinical setting (e.g. most first AVM-related haemorrhages occur before age 35–40) and radiographic

Table 6.1 Boston criteria for CAA-related haemorrhage

	Classic Boston criteria
Definite CAA	Full post-mortem examination demonstrating:
	lobar, cortical, or cortico-subcortical haemorrhage
	severe CAA with vasculopathy
	absence of other diagnostic lesion
Probable CAA with supporting pathology	Clinical data and pathological tissue (evacuated haematoma or cortical biopsy) demonstrating:
	lobar, cortical, or cortico-subcortical haemorrhage
	some degree of CAA in specimen
	absence of other diagnostic lesion
Probable CAA	Clinical data and MRI or CT demonstrating:
	multiple haemorrhages restricted to lobar, cortical, or cortico-subcortical regions (cerebellar haemorrhage allowed)
	age ≥55 years
	absence of other cause of haemorrhage
Possible CAA	Clinical data and MRI or CT demonstrating:
	single lobar, cortical, or cortico-subcortical haemorrhage
	age ≥55 years
	absence of other cause of haemorrhage

appearance. Gradient echo MRI can be helpful in this regard by establishing the presence and distribution of previous haemorrhages. Another helpful study is a follow-up MRI performed 2–3 months after the primary haemorrhage to rule out an underlying vascular malformation or tumour.

Multiple haemorrhages can be seen with CNS vasculitis (see Cases 11, 15, and 25), hypertensive encephalopathy, multiple cavernous malformations (see Case 44), or coagulopathy. These conditions generally can be distinguished from CAA by the clinical setting and distribution of haemorrhages, which typically do not follow the same anatomical pattern as CAA (restriction to cortical or grey–white regions) (see Case 40).

CAA is defined by the deposition of amyloid in the walls of leptomeningeal and cortical arteries, arterioles, capillaries, and veins. This CNS vasculopathy is associated with a number of clinical sydromes including recurrent lobar haemorrhage, subcortical ischaemia, migraine, and dementia. CAA may be hereditary or sporadic. Hereditary forms, mostly associated with amyloid precursor protein mutations, are rare, but the sporadic form increases exponentially with age. It is rare before the age of 50 years and common in 90-year-olds. Clinical presentations of CAA include the following:

Lobar haemorrhage

The lobar location of the haemorrhages reflects the underlying distribution of the vascular amyloid deposits which has a predilection for cortical vessels and largely spares white matter, deep grey matter, and the brainstem. The reason for higher rates of CAA-related haemorrhage in the posterior brain is unclear, but it may be related to as yet unknown characteristics of posterior circulation vessels that influence β-amyloid peptide elimination, or to increased vulnerability of these brain regions to minor trauma.

The haematoma commonly involves the cortico-subcortical region, particularly of the frontal or occipital lobes, and may extend into the subarachnoid space or the ventricles. The term 'lobar' refers to location in the cortex and subcortical white matter in contrast to the deep brain locations (putamen, thalamus, and pons) characteristic of hypertensive haemorrhage. CAA-related haemorrhages tend to cluster in posterior brain regions and within the same lobe in a given individual. Recurrent lobar haemorrhage is the most overt syndrome associated with CAA and accounts for 5–20% of all spontaneous (non-traumatic) cerebral haemorrhages in elderly subjects. Recurrent haemorrhage is more likely with increasing number of microhaemorrhages and with posterior white matter hypodensity on CT scan which may be markers of severity of underlying CAA.

Cerebral ischaemia

CAA is associated to a lesser extent with small ischaemic lesions, usually located in the cerebral cortex. These may present as TIA or minor stroke. The aetiology is unclear.

Subarachnoid haemorrhage (SAH)

SAH may occur and is frequently cortical although it may be secondary in large parenchymal haemorrhage. Localized cortical haemorrhage is thought to occur from rupture of the meningo-cortical vessels.

Leukoaraiosis

Diffuse white matter damage occurs in hereditary forms of CAA, and in sporadic CAA there is often periventricular leukoaraiosis in which demyelination, gliosis, and incomplete infarction are present (see Case 49).

Transient neurological symptoms

Transient neurological symptoms are a less common but clinically important manifestation of CAA. Patients complain of recurrent, brief (minutes), often stereotyped spells of weakness, numbness, paraesthesiae, or other cortical symptoms that can spread smoothly over contiguous body parts. These episodes may reflect abnormal activity (either focal seizure or spreading depression) of the surrounding cortex in response to small haemorrhages. There are anecdotal observations that anticonvulsants may stop the attacks. Features that help distinguish these spells from true TIAs include the smooth spread of the symptoms, the absence of haemodynamically significant stenosis in the relevant vascular supply, and the presence of small haemorrhages in the corresponding region of cortex.

Dementia

The relationship between CAA and cognitive impairment and dementia is well recognized. In neuropathological series, increasing CAA is associated with poorer cognitive performance and there is frequently associated Alzheimer's disease (AD) pathology. The mechanisms of cognitive impairment include ischaemic or haemorrhagic stroke, causing cognitive impairment through strategic effects or disruption of multiple cerebral circuits (see Case 8), interference with cerebral autoregulation with secondary white matter ischaemia, and inhibition of blood–brain barrier transport caused by amyloid deposition. These patients can present with progressive dementia reminiscent of subcortical arteriosclerotic encephalopathy (Binswanger's disease—see Case 49). The distributions of white matter changes in CAA and in hypertensive vasculopathy appear to be similar.

As with cognitive impairment and dementia in general, there is variation in cognitive performance for a given degree of abnormality on brain imaging: some patients with severe white matter change and microbleeds may be cognitively normal, whereas others with similar changes may be demented. This is illustrated in the three cases discussed here, where Case 6.A showed severe changes on imaging but had normal cognitive function whereas Case 6.C, with less dramatic imaging findings, had dementia. However, in general, severe white matter change is associated with cognitive decline that manifests particularly in executive and motivational deficits and decreases in motor speed (see Case 49).

Rarely, CAA is associated with a rapid cognitive decline. In such cases, there appears to be an inflammatory vasculitis with multinucleated giant cells in vessel walls and macrophages with internalized amyloid. Rapid cognitive decline may be seen, particularly in the domains of language and praxis, and there may be seizures and hallucinations.

3. What advice would you give regarding medication?

There are few data to guide therapeutic decisions in patients with CAA.

Antithrombotic agents

Antithrombotic agents appear to increase the risk of recurrent haemorrhage in CAA.

- ◆ Warfarin appears to increase both the frequency and severity of cerebral haemorrhage and should be avoided, if possible, in patients with CAA.

- ◆ Aspirin at commonly prescribed doses increases the risk of haemorrhage to a lesser extent. In one prospective cohort of patients with primary lobar intracerebral haemorrhage (ICH), aspirin was associated with an increased risk of ICH recurrence (HR = 3.95; 95% CI 1.6–8.3) when controlling for other haemorrhage risk factors. Nonetheless, aspirin use can be considered in selected patients with CAA if they have clear indications for antiplatelet therapy.

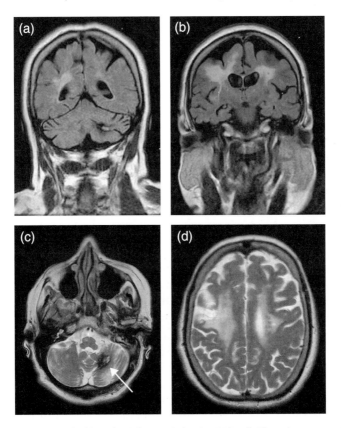

Fig. 6.5 Coronal FLAIR (a, b) and axial T2-weighted MRI (c, d). There is an area of haemosiderin staining inferiorly in the left cerebellar hemisphere in the region of the previous left cerebellar haematoma (arrow) (c). There is extensive small vessel ischaemic change (a, b, d).

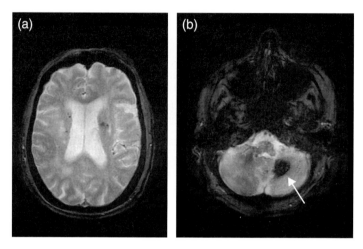

Fig. 6.6 GRE MR sequences showing multiple microhaemorrhages and the old left cerebellar haemorrhage (arrow).

Figures 6.5 and 6.6 show the MRI brain scans from a patient with a past history of cerebellar haemorrhage and subsequent recurrent ischaemic stroke and AF. Warfarin was not given owing to her previous haemorrhage and the presence of microbleeds, and thus a likely increased risk of further ICH. The images show an area of haemosiderin staining inferiorly in the left cerebellar hemisphere in the region of the previous left cerebellar haematoma (Fig. 6.5(c)). There is extensive small vessel ischaemic change (Figs 6.5(a), 6.5(b) and 6.5(d)). The gradient echo sequences (Fig. 6.6) show multiple microhaemorrhages in both hemispheres and a larger bleed in the left cerebellar hemisphere.

Blood pressure control

Although the vascular pathology in CAA does not appear to be linked to hypertension, control of blood pressure is nonetheless advisable. Support for lowering of blood pressure in patients diagnosed with CAA came from a secondary analysis of data from the PROGRESS trial. Randomization to active treatment (perindopril plus indapamide) resulted in a 77% reduction in the risk of probable CAA-related ICH.

Further reading

Biffi, A, Halpin, A, Towfighi, A, *et al.* (2010). Aspirin and recurrent intracerebral hemorrhage in cerebral amyloid angiopathy. *Neurology*; **75**: 693–8.

Greenberg, SM, Eng, JA, Ning, M, *et al.* (2004) Hemorrhage burden predicts recurrent intracerebral hemorrhage after lobar hemorrhage. *Stroke*; **35**:1415–20.

Greenberg SM, Gurol ME, Rosand J, Smith EE. (2004). Amyloid angiopathy-related vascular cognitive impairment. *Stroke*; **35**(Suppl 1): 2616–19.

Knudsen KA, Rosand J, Karluk D, Greenberg SM (2001). Clinical diagnosis of cerebral amyloid angiopathy: validation of the Boston criteria. *Neurology*; **56**: 537–9.

Maia LF, Mackenzie IR, Feldman HH (2007). Clinical phenotypes of cerebral amyloid angiopathy. *J Neurol Sci*; **257**: 23–30.

Smith EE, Eichler F (2006). Cerebral amyloid angiopathy and lobar intracerebral hemorrhage. *Arch Neurol*; **63**: 148–51.

Case 7

Case 7.A

A 65-year-old woman presented with three episodes of left-sided visual disturbance. She described 'looking through broken glass', which persisted for 10 minutes. She was unsure how quickly the visual disturbance came on and whether it affected her left eye or left visual field. Shortly after the visual disturbance the patient developed a severe throbbing headache associated with nausea, which persisted for several hours. The patient had a history of hypertension, for which she had been prescribed a Ca antagonist. She had stopped smoking 6 months previously (10–15 cigarettes per day for at least 40 years). She had never been prone to headache before.

Investigations showed the following:
- MRI brain: scattered small vessel disease; no recent infarction
- MRA: 95% stenosis of the left ICA

Case 7.B

A 45-year-old woman with a long history of migraine with visual aura presented with a 3-day history of a right hemianopia and right-sided sensory disturbance. She usually had one or two migraine attacks per month. Her usual attacks started with seeing flashing lights and subsequent right-sided visual loss. She also very frequently developed paraesthesiae and numbness spreading over the right side of her face and right arm. These symptoms were followed by a unilateral headache (usually left-sided). The neurological disturbance normally lasted up to 2 hours, with the headache persisting for 6–12 hours. On this occasion, the patient developed her usual visual and sensory disturbance and headache, but she was worried that, although the headache had disappeared, her visual and sensory symptoms still persisted 3 days after symptom onset. The patient was otherwise well with no previous medical problems. She denied any history of hypertension, diabetes, or heart disease. She had never smoked. Her father had had migraine, but otherwise there was no family history of note.

Investigations showed the following:
- MRI brain: recent left occipital infarct
- MRA of cervical and intracranial vessels: normal
- ECG, 24-hour tape, transthoracic and transoesophageal echocardiogram, thrombophilia screen, auto-antibody screen, cholesterol, glucose: all normal.

Case 7.C

A 50-year-old man with a long history of recurrent migrainous headache presented to the TIA clinic. He had developed a fairly rapid onset sensory disturbance and weakness of his right arm, although he described that he had first been aware of symptoms in his right hand, but that over the next 1–2 minutes the symptoms had spread to involve the entire arm. The patient also became aware of a numb feeling affecting the right side of his face and had difficulty speaking—he described this as not being able to say what he wanted. These symptoms persisted for about an hour and were followed by the patient's usual migraine headache. However, he denied ever having experienced any focal symptoms with previous migraine attacks, although he recalled that his mother had difficulty speaking when she had a severe migraine attack. The patient himself had a history of smoking a cigar every evening, and he had a raised cholesterol level.

Investigations showed the following:

◆ MRI brain and MRA of cervical and intracranial vessels: normal
◆ ECG and 24-hour tape: normal
◆ Echocardiogram: normal
◆ Cholesterol: 6.3mmol/L
◆ Random glucose: 5.7mmol/L.

Questions

1. All these patients represent a common diagnostic dilemma. What are the two main diagnostic categories?
2. What is the diagnosis in each patient?
3. Discuss clinical features in the history which may help you to differentiate between the two main possible diagnoses in Case 7.C.

Answers

1. All these patients represent a common diagnostic dilemma. What are the two main diagnostic categories?

All these cases demonstrate the complex relationship between cerebral ischaemic events and migraine. Migraine can mimic cerebral ischaemic events, migraine is a risk factor for stroke, migraine can cause a stroke, a TIA or stroke may present as migraine, and finally some disorders, such as CADASIL or antiphospholipid syndrome, may present with both migraine and stroke. These multiple associations are summarized in Table 7.1. While these associations are well recognized, the underlying mechanisms are less clear, and we will discuss them in more detail with individual cases in this and other chapters.

2. What is the diagnosis in each patient?

Case 7.A. Migraine as a symptom of underlying ischaemia

This patient describes migraine with visual aura. While a first migraine attack can occur at any age, the most common age of onset is 20–40 years, and any later onset should cause suspicion of an underlying disorder. This woman has a severe ICA stenosis, which is a recognized cause of symptomatic migraine. In addition to atheromatous disease, migrainous symptoms have more commonly been described in cervical (carotid and vertebral) artery dissection and arteriovenous malformations. Therefore new-onset migraine, in particular in elderly patients and in patients with vascular risk factors, requires a full assessment for vascular disease. Neurological assessment and brain and vascular imaging are indicated even in younger patients if they present with a new onset of migraine, usually with aura, or with a change in frequency or character of previous migraine symptoms.

Table 7.1 Associations of migraine with stroke

Migraine as a cause of stroke	Migrainous infarction
Migraine as a risk factor for stroke	Migraine may be a risk factor for stroke in the presence of other risk factors, e.g. in combination with use of the oral contraceptive pill and smoking in young women
Migraine as a symptom of ischaemia	Carotid stenosis or arteriovenous malformation causing migrainous symptoms
Coexisting stroke and migraine	Stroke and migraine are common conditions and may coexist in some patients without being otherwise associated
Clinical presentation of underlying condition includes both migraine and stroke	Examples: CADASIL or antiphospholipid syndrome

How vascular disease causes migrainous symptoms is poorly understood. Migrainous aura is caused by cortical spreading depression. This has also been demonstrated in ischaemic stroke, and it has been suggested that ischaemia causes cortical spreading depression. In severe carotid stenosis, there may be underlying chronic ischaemia which acts as a trigger for cortical spreading depression. Similarly, in arteriovenous malformations changes in blood flow may cause ischaemia. Interestingly, migrainous symptoms, in particular unilateral headache, have been described more frequently in posterior circulation events. In our current patient, migrainous symptoms arose from an impaired anterior circulation. The patient underwent carotid endarterectomy a week after her original assessment. Two months after the procedure, she was symptom free and had had no further migrainous episodes.

Case 7.B. Migrainous infarction

This woman has an infarction corresponding to the area of the brain from which her aura symptoms arise. She experienced one of her typical auras at the onset of her stroke, and detailed investigation for possible causes of stroke have not brought up any other possible aetiology for her stroke. This woman fulfils the criteria for migrainous infarction.

Although the International Headache Society now recognize migrainous infarction as an entity, the mechanism of how migraine causes a stroke is poorly understood. Several studies have shown that the cortical spreading depression during a migraine attack is followed by a similar wave of hypoperfusion. However, it is still not clear if this hypoperfusion can become sufficiently severe to cause infarction. Other mechanisms suggested for migrainous stroke include vasospasm or hypercoagulability caused by the release of inflammatory mediators.

Case 7.C. Migraine as a TIA mimic

This patient represents a very common diagnostic dilemma in TIA clinics: he has a history of migraine, but he also has several vascular risk factors. He now presents with an episode that sounds migrainous in character, but is different from his previous attacks and could also have been ischaemic in nature. Some features in the history may help to differentiate between migraine with aura and a TIA (see Table 7.2). Unfortunately, the history is often far less clear cut, and there are no investigations which can differentiate between TIA and migraine with certainty.

Given the change of character in the migraine attack in this patient, in that he now had focal symptoms in addition to his usual headache, further investigation is indicated. If any underlying structural lesion is found, it should be treated accordingly. Any vascular risk factors warrant treatment in their own right. However, making a diagnosis of cerebral ischaemic event versus migraine can potentially have far-reaching consequences in terms of employment (e.g. professional driving), insurance, and taking long-term secondary preventative medication. The only advice is to take the history with care and perhaps repeatedly, and, in management, to find the right balance between sufficient secondary prevention and having as little impact as possible on the patient's life, and this will clearly depend on individual circumstances.

Table 7.2 Features which may help to distinguish between migraine aura and TIA

Migraine aura	Transient ischaemic attack	Comments
Gradual onset over seconds to minutes	Rapid sudden onset	
Symptoms may spread, e.g. paraesthesiae spreading from the hand to involve the whole arm	All symptoms present straight away	
'Positive' symptoms, i.e. paraesthesiae, flashing lights	'Negative symptoms', i.e. sensory loss, visual loss	
Aura symptoms frequently followed by unilateral throbbing headache	Headache occurs less frequently	Headache can occur in stroke/TIA, especially in posterior circulation events.
Prior history of migraine, perhaps even similar attacks		20% of the population have migraine at some point—not a reliable distinguishing feature

3. Discuss clinical features in the history which may help you to differentiate between the two main possible diagnoses in Case 7.C.

Features which may help differentiate between an attack of migraine and a TIA are listed in Table 7.2. However, it is important to recognize that no single feature can differentiate reliably between these two conditions. Migraine aura can be of sudden onset, patients with sensory TIAs may experience positive symptoms, and, of course, migrainous symptoms in themselves may be caused by ischaemia. Quite often it will be impossible to decide if a patient has had one or the other, and further management will be very much an individual decision.

Further reading

Bousser MG, Welch KMA (2005). Relation between migraine and stroke. *Lancet Neurol*; **4**: 533–42.

Weinberger J (2006). Interactions between migraine and stroke. *Curr Treat Options Neurol*; **8**: 513–17.

Case 8

An 82-year-old man, who was living alone, was referred to the acute medical take from the emergency department. He had fallen and sustained a Colles fracture of the right forearm. He had been assessed by the occupational therapist in the emergency department and it had been decided that he could not be discharged home without care. He had a past history of two strokes in the previous 12 months, the most recent occurring 3 months prior to admission. He had apparently made a good recovery and had returned to his flat. Regular medication included amlodipine, bendroflumethiazide, aspirin, and simvastatin.

When interviewed by the medical team, he was able to give a reasonable account of events leading up to admission although he was vague about specific dates and times. His son felt that he had not been coping well on his own at home and had suffered frequent falls. On examination, the pulse was 70bpm and regular, but blood pressure was 100/70mmHg lying falling to 70/30mmHg standing. Neurological examination showed an upgoing left plantar reflex but was otherwise normal.

On the medical ward, he was mobile and able to wash and dress independently but was intermittently incontinent of urine and faeces, although this did not seem to trouble him.

CT brain is shown in Figure 8.1.

Questions

1. In view of the clinical features of the case, the occupational therapist's report, and the son's information, what further clinical examination should be performed and which test might you choose?

2. What would you expect your further testing to show? Why has the patient developed this problem?

3. How would you manage this case?

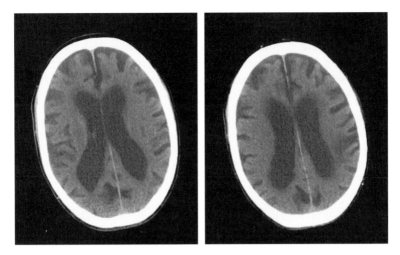

Fig. 8.1 CT brain.

Answers

1. In view of the clinical features of the case, the occupational therapist's report, and the son's information, what further clinical examination should be performed and which test might you choose?

Cognitive testing should be performed.

The history of failure to cope at home and incontinence, about which the patient appears unconcerned, suggest the possibility of cognitive impairment. In this case, the patient had a Mini-Mental State Examination (MMSE) score of 24/30 and a Montreal Cognitive Assessment (MoCA) score of 18/30 consistent with impaired cognition.

There is no consensus about which short screening tests of global cognition are best. The MMSE is relatively insensitive to milder cognitive impairments, in particular frontal lobe/executive deficits, since it does not contain items that test these domains. In early vascular cognitive impairment, frontal (executive and attentional) deficits are often prominent compared with early Alzheimer type impairment in which short-term memory deficits are more apparent (although many patients have overlapping pathology and hence overlapping clinical characteristics). Thus patients with vascular cognitive impairment, in particular, may perform reasonably well on the MMSE despite significant deficits, and further cognitive testing should be considered.

The MoCA was recently developed to distinguish between normal cognition and mild cognitive impairment and, like the MMSE, is a 30-point score. However, the MoCA allocates 5 of 30 possible points for visuospatial/executive tasks, whereas the MMSE is strongly weighted towards memory (6/30 points) and orientation (10/30 points). The MoCA has been shown to be a reliable measure of cognition in subjects with Alzheimer-type cognitive decline, Parkinson's disease, and cerebrovascular disease. Another frequently used global screen is the Addenbrooke's Cognitive Examination Revised (ACE-R), a 100-point score that contains the MMSE embedded within it. The ACE-R also contains visuo-executive tasks and appears valid in cerebro-vascular disease. It contains many language items, reflecting the fact that it was developed in part for the assessment of frontotemporal dementia.

2. What would you expect your further testing to show? Why has the patient developed this problem?

This patient has post-stroke dementia.

This patient has several factors that are associated with cognitive impairment in addition to his age. Probably the most important is the fact that he has suffered two recent strokes. The CT scan shows atrophy and evidence of his previous left frontoparietal infarct. Stroke is a risk factor for dementia, and having a stroke brings forward the onset of dementia by around 10 years. A meta-analysis of studies of the prevalence of post-stroke dementia showed that over 90% of the variance between studies in reported rates of post-stroke dementia could be explained by three study factors: inclusion/exclusion of patients demented prior to stroke (pre-stroke dementia), inclusion of first ever stroke only versus recurrent stroke, and whether the study was population- or hospital-based. When the available data were stratified according to these three factors, there was good agreement between studies, and pooled analysis showed that in hospital-based studies of patients with recurrent stroke, over 30% had dementia in the first year after stroke.

Individual studies and pooled longitudinal data show a steep rise in dementia incidence in the first few months after stroke. Thereafter rates are lower and would be lower still in the absence of recurrent stroke. The mechanism by which stroke causes dementia is unclear. There may be unmasking of pre-existing degenerative pathology, and in support of this pre-stroke cognitive decline is a risk factor for post-stroke dementia. Alternatively, the stroke may precipitate acceleration of existing degenerative change. Finally, the occurrence of stroke may combine with previous stroke or white matter disease (see Case 49) to cause functional disconnection of trans-cerebral circuits. Although hypertension is a risk factor for stroke and dementia, it is not more common in those with stroke who develop dementia than in those remaining undemented. Regarding stroke subtype there is some evidence that haemorrhagic stroke is associated with greater dementia risk than ischaemic stroke perhaps through greater stroke severity or because of associations with underlying CAA (see Case 6). Dementia incidence rates are lower in population-based studies than in hospital-based studies because of the inclusion of first ever stroke only and more minor cerebrovascular events in population-based studies. Females are slightly more likely than males to develop post-stroke dementia, but female sex is a stronger risk factor for pre-stroke dementia.

Factors associated with the development of post-stroke dementia include prior cognitive impairment, the presence of multiple lesions, AF, diabetes, hypotension/hypoxia, seizures and urinary incontinence in the acute post-stroke period, and the presence of cerebral atrophy and white matter disease. Secondary insults are known to be important in adverse cognitive outcome after head injury, and aggressive treatment to maintain physiological homeostasis after stroke may well improve cognitive outcome. Low education is also associated, as it is for all causes of dementia. Many of the factors associated with pre-stroke dementia are similar to those for post-stroke dementia. However, there are important differences in the strength of certain factor associations between pre- and post-stroke dementia. Age, medial temporal lobe atrophy, family history, and female sex are all more strongly associated with pre-stroke dementia, suggesting a more important role for degenerative pathology in pre-stroke compared with post-stroke dementia.

Hypertension in mid-life is a risk factor for the development of subsequent dementia. However, it is less clear whether development of hypertension in later life is similarly predictive beyond its being a risk factor for stroke. It also remains unclear whether treatment of hypertension after a stroke has any impact on the risk of subsequent cognitive decline beyond reducing stroke risk. Hypotension in the immediate post-stroke phase is deleterious to cognition, and it is possible that this was a factor in this man's cognitive decline. The presence of urinary incontinence in the immediate post-stroke period may be significant since this is associated with post-stroke dementia, possibly through a link to stroke severity or as an indicator of frontal lobe damage.

3. How would you manage this case?

Management includes the following:

- the diagnosis of dementia should be explained
- antihypertensives should be stopped
- causes of incontinence should be sought
- full occupational therapy (OT) assessment is required.

It is important that the diagnosis of dementia is explained to the patient and his family. Early dementia diagnosis enables the patient to make decisions about future care and to consider lasting power of attorney with his family; it is possible that he retains the capacity to decide whether he wishes to give the control of his financial affairs and decisions regarding his medical care to a close family member once he loses capacity.

There are some data to suggest that earlier dementia diagnosis is associated with increased time to institutionalization and reduced crisis admissions.

The antihypertensive medication should be stopped since it is causing the patient to have falls and is likely to exacerbate his cognitive disability. There is some suggestion that postural hypotension is linked to increased blood pressure variability, and that these two factors are associated with vascular dementia.

Causes of incontinence should be sought including:

- urinary tract infection and constipation
- bladder outflow tract obstruction
- lack of ability to find the toilet.

This patient requires further OT assessment with respect to his home situation. He is likely to return home with care (rather than be admitted to a care home) and with follow-up from the psychogeriatrics–dementia team. In terms of pharmacotherapy, there is little evidence to support the use of cholinesterase inhibitors in patients with vascular cognitive impairment. Maintaining an active life where possible, including attending a day centre with the opportunity to socialize, may help maintain cognitive function.

Further reading

Dong Y, Sharma VK, Chan BP, *et al.* (2010). The Montreal Cognitive Assessment (MoCA) is superior to the Mini-Mental State Examination (MMSE) for the detection of vascular cognitive impairment after acute stroke. *J Neurol Sci*; **299**: 15–18.

Mioshi E, Dawson K, Mitchell J, Arnold R, Hodges JR (2006). The Addenbrooke's Cognitive Examination Revised (ACE-R): a brief cognitive test battery for dementia screening. *Int J Geriatr Psychiatry*; **21**: 1078–85.

Nasreddine ZS, Phillips NA, Bedirian V, *et al.* (2005) The Montreal Cognitive Assessment, MoCA: a brief screening tool for mild cognitive impairment. *J Am Geriatr Soc*; **53**: 695–9.

Pendlebury ST, Rothwell PM (2009). Prevalence, incidence, and factors associated with pre-stroke and post-stroke dementia: a systematic review and meta-analysis. *Lancet Neurol*; **8**: 1006–18.

Pendlebury ST, Cuthbertson FC, Welch SJ, Mehta Z, Rothwell PM (2010). Underestimation of cognitive impairment by Mini-Mental State Examination versus the Montreal Cognitive Assessment in patients with transient ischemic attack and stroke: a population-based study. *Stroke*; **41**: 1290–3.

Pendlebury ST, Mariz J, Bull LM, *et al.* (in press). Montreal Cognitive Assessment, Addenbrooke's cognitive examination-revised and mini-mental state examination versus the NINDS-CSN vascular cognitive impairment neuropsychological battery in patients with TIA and stroke. *Stroke.*

De Ronchi D, Palmer K, Pioggiosi P, *et al.* (2007). The combined effect of age, education, and stroke on dementia and cognitive impairment/no dementia in the elderly. *Dement Geriatr Cogn Disord*; **24**: 266–73.

Case 9

A 40-year-old car salesman was admitted to the local stroke unit after having woken with dysarthria and unsteadiness. He had been feeling non-specifically unwell and had some blurred vision the day before. The next day he developed diplopia, mild dysphagia, and paraesthesiae in hands and feet. He also became increasingly drowsy. He had recently returned from a holiday in the Canary Islands, where he had had some diarrhoea and vomiting 2 weeks prior to presentation. Otherwise, there was no past history of note. The patient was a non-smoker and denied any illicit drug use.

On examination the patient was drowsy, but rousable and appropriate. He was dysarthric and had a complete internal and external ophthalmoplegia with bilateral ptosis but no facial weakness. There was mild bilateral arm weakness but full power in the legs and marked truncal and gait ataxia exceeding the degree of limb weakness. The reflexes were symmetrically brisk with bilateral extensor plantar responses. There was no sensory deficit.

Questions

1. Do you think that this patient has had a vascular event? What is your differential diagnosis?
2. Which investigations would you do next?
3. How would you treat this patient?

Answers

1. Do you think that this patient has had a vascular event? What is your differential diagnosis?

The patient awoke with neurological symptoms. This suggests a rapid, if not sudden, symptom onset which might be in keeping with a vascular aetiology. However, the history suggests that the patient was already feeling unwell the day before, and his symptoms progressed over subsequent days. Overall, the history suggests rapidly progressive symptoms, but there is no clear evidence of a sudden or stepwise deterioration. While not impossible, this type of symptom progression would be unusual for a vascular event. Other diagnostic possibilities include an inflammatory process due to an infectious, para-infectious, or autoimmune aetiology. Symptom onset appears too rapid for a tumour, although this may occasionally occur (see Case 1).

The patient's symptoms and signs point towards the middle and upper brainstem being affected by the disease process. Drowsiness can arise from the reticular formation (pons) being affected, and the ophthalmoplegia equally suggests a pontine and lower midbrain lesion. The ataxia suggests bilateral involvement of the cerebellar tracts, and the mild weakness some involvement of the pyramidal tracts/anterior brainstem. Lack of a sensory deficit suggests that the posterior brainstem is relatively spared. Overall, there appears to be quite widespread brainstem involvement which does not conform to a specific vascular territory and would therefore make an ischaemic event unlikely. Furthermore, if such a widespread brainstem area had been affected by ischaemia or haemorrhage, one would expect the patient to be much more unwell as these would cause severe structural damage. In this patient, even though there appears to be widespread brainstem involvement, function seems to be impaired rather than completely abolished. This would be more in keeping with an inflammatory process rather than a vascular event.

Symptom progression in this patient is therefore most in keeping with an inflammatory process affecting the mid- and upper brainstem. The temporal association with a diarrhoeal illness 2 weeks previously would suggest an infectious or para-infectious process. A further possibility may be a metabolic cause, such as central pontine myelinolysis or Wernicke's encephalopathy. However, there is nothing in the history to suggest that the diarrhoeal illness was sufficiently severe to cause significant metabolic derangement. Finally, the diarrhoeal illness may, of course, have been entirely unrelated and the symptoms could be due to an autoimmune process, such as multiple sclerosis. Although there are a large number of diagnostic possibilities, the clinical presentation is typical of Bickerstaff brainstem encephalitis (BBE). This is a post-infectious encephalitis, in which patients typically present with a combination of ophthalmoplegia, ataxia, and reduced level of consciousness or long tract signs.

2. Which investigations would you do next?

Further investigation should be directed towards confirming the clinical diagnosis, finding the underlying aetiology, and excluding other diagnoses.

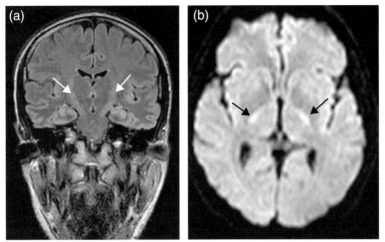

Fig. 9.1 MRI brain: (a) coronal FLAIR image; (b) axial diffusion-weighted image. Symmetrical hyperintensity of the corticospinal tract at the level of the brainstem and medulla, with possibly restricted diffusion in the corticospinal tracts on DWI (arrows).

In this patient the brainstem appears to be the affected structure. The next step is to proceed to imaging to try and define the underlying pathological process further. This is best done with MRI, as CT of the posterior fossa and brainstem is susceptible to artefacts from the surrounding bone. Further investigations depend on the imaging results. The patient's scan is shown in Fig. 9.1. MRI brain shows symmetrical hyperintensity of the corticospinal tract at the level of the brainstem and medulla, with possibly restricted diffusion on DWI. Although sometimes seen in healthy individuals, in this patient the appearances were felt to be in keeping with the clinically suspected inflammatory brainstem process, and they were also in keeping with a diagnosis of BBE, in which high-signal lesions affecting the brainstem, thalamus, cerebellum, and cerebrum are found in up to a third of patients.

BBE is frequently associated with antiganglioside antibodies, in particular with anti-GQ1b antibodies. These should be looked for in serological studies. Furthermore, the CSF in BBE may be abnormal: protein is elevated in about half of patients, and a third of patients will have a raised white cell count (WCC). In addition to substantiating the diagnosis of BBE further, CSF and blood should also be studied to rule out any other diagnosis (e.g. direct CNS infection). Furthermore, if a diagnosis of BBE is confirmed, it may also still be possible to identify the underlying causative infectious agent. Therefore CSF should be sent for culture, viral polymerase chain reactions (PCRs), viral serologies (specifically HSV, JC virus), listeria, oligoclonal bands, cytology, and perhaps angiotensin-converting enzyme (ACE). Concurrent blood tests should include anti-ganglioside antibodies, especially anti-GQ1b antibodies, autoantibodies, serum electrophoresis for parallel testing with CSF for oligoclonal bands, viral serologies including HIV testing, *Listeria*, *Campylobacter*, and *Mycoplasma*.

Patients should have a CXR to look for an associated atypical pneumonia or possibly neoplasm causing a paraneoplastic process.

In this patient, CSF examination showed acellular fluid and normal glucose, but a raised protein of 1.5g/dl. Serological tests were positive for Campylobacter IgM, which was suggestive of a recent infection. Anti-GM1 antibodies were positive. Given the history of the preceding illness, the imaging findings of high signal in the brainstem, the albumin–cytological dissociation in the CSF, the serological findings of a recent Campylobacter infection and the presence of anti-ganglioside antibodies, a diagnosis of BBE was made.

3. How would you treat this patient?

BBE is often regarded as part of the Miller–Fisher syndrome or Guillain–Barré syndrome spectrum of disorders. Like these, it usually occurs after an infection and is associated with the presence of anti-ganglioside antibodies. Given this overlap, a similar treatment approach would be logical. Patients have been treated with a variety of immunomodulating therapies, such as intravenous human immunoglobulin, plasma exchange, or steroids. No trial data are available to determine the efficacy of these different approaches. Moreover, the prognosis of BBE is generally good. Almost all patients have a monophasic remitting course of their illness, and at 6 months two-thirds of patients have made a full recovery. In such a generally benign illness it is difficult to be certain of the benefit of any therapeutic intervention.

It may be more difficult to decide how to treat this patient before the diagnosis is established. In particular, the initial differential diagnosis also included infectious viral encephalitis. While the presentation would be unusual for herpes simplex encephalitis, this can also affect the brainstem, and, if not treated, may potentially result in severe disability or death. Therefore, if there are no clear contraindications, such patients should be treated with aciclovir until the results of viral PCR studies are available.

Further reading

Odaka M, Yuki N, Yamada M, *et al.* (2003). Bickerstaff's brainstem encephalitis: clinical features of 62 cases and a subgroup associated with Guillain–Barré syndrome. *Brain*; **126**: 2279–90.

Overell JR, Willison HJ (2005). Recent developments in Miller–Fisher syndrome and associated disorders. *Curr Opin Neurol*; **18**: 562–6.

Case 10

A 74-year-old man was referred to the emergency TIA clinic with an episode of sudden onset of word-finding difficulty accompanied by right arm weakness that had gradually resolved after a couple of days. At the time of this event, he also reported some pain and difficulty using his left leg that had also gradually improved. The patient was not certain whether the left leg had been weak rather than just painful. There was a past history of type 2 diabetes and hypertension for which he was on treatment. On examination, pulse was regular, blood pressure was 145/85mmHg, and heart sounds were normal. There was slight hesitancy of speech and minor word-finding difficulties together with an extensor right plantar response.

Investigations showed the following:

◆ ECG: sinus rhythm and left ventricular hypertrophy by voltage
◆ CXR: no evidence of cardiomegaly
◆ CT brain excluded a bleed but showed no definite area of infarction that could explain his symptoms
◆ Carotid Doppler showed an occlusion of the left internal carotid artery and an 85% stenosis of the right ICA.

Question

1. Would you refer this man for carotid endarterectomy?

Answer

1. Would you refer this man for carotid endarterectomy?

The management of this patient is not straightforward. His presentation with dysphasia and right arm weakness indicates a TIA in the left MCA territory, but his concurrent left leg weakness suggests that his right hemisphere may also have been affected.

There are several possible explanations for this patient's bihemispheric symptoms. Cardiac emboli are a possibility, although unlikely, as the left carotid artery is occluded and therefore would not allow any emboli to pass. The TIAs may be of haemodynamic origin, given that this patient has severe bilateral carotid occlusive disease. However, the absence of any postural component to his symptoms perhaps makes this less likely. Finally, emboli from the right internal carotid artery stenosis may also pass over to the left hemisphere via collateral flow through the Circle of Willis.

Carotid endarterectomy is indicated in the presence of a recently symptomatic stenosis of 70-99%, with surgery also being considered in some patients with 50-69% stenosis, for example in men, very early presentation and the presence of plaque ulceration. Surgery is not offered to patients with carotid occlusion, as there is no flow distal to the occlusion and thus no risk of embolization. In the current patient, the difficulty was to decide if he had been symptomatic from his right ICA-stenosis, and therefore if he should have a right carotid endarterectomy. In the end it was decided to proceed with right carotid endarterectomy, because regardless of whether the left hemispheric symptoms were due to low flow or embolization via the Circle of Willis, the risk of further events from either aetiology would be reduced with right carotid surgery.

Whilst awaiting surgery, the patient was treated with antiplatelet drugs and a statin, but not with antihypertensive agents. This was to ensure adequate blood flow through his stenosed vessels. Nevertheless, prior to surgery he unfortunately had a further event resulting in mild dysphasia. MRI showed an acute infarct in the left cerebral cortex (Fig. 10.1) and repeat carotid Dopplers at this stage suggested there was some trickle flow in the left internal carotid artery. However, this was not confirmed by the MRA (Fig. 10.2), which still showed a left ICA occlusion.

There was some debate if further more invasive vascular imaging was indicated to see if the patient had a left carotid near-occlusion with some residual flow or a complete carotid occlusion, and whether left carotid surgery would be indicated. However, even in the presence of trickle flow, the risk of stroke distal to a near-occlusion is low, and the feeling was that this patient's prognosis was more likely to be improved by proceeding with right-sided endarterectomy to increase blood flow and to reduce the risk of further embolic events. The patient underwent surgery, and he was well six months after the operation, with no further episodes of ischaemia, although he still had some residual hesitancy of speech and word finding difficulties.

In the pooled analysis of the trials of carotid endarterectomy, it was shown that stenosed vessels with post-stenotic collapse or 'near occlusions' had a very low

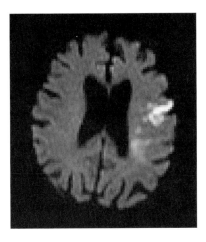

Fig. 10.1 DWI shows an acute infarct in the left cerebral cortex.

risk of stroke on follow up and thus the risks of surgery outweighed the benefits. The low risk of stroke is most likely due to the presence of a good colateral circulation, which is visible on angiography in the vast majority of the patients with narrowing of the ICA distal to a severe stenosis. Some patients with near occlusion

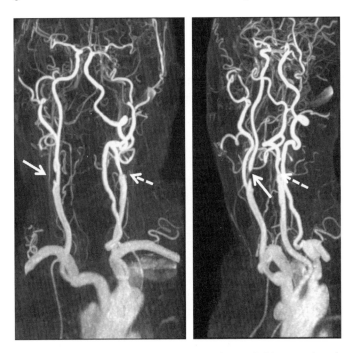

Fig. 10.2 The MRA shows a severe stenosis of the right ICA (white arrow) and an occluded left ICA (white dashed arrow). The right vertebral artery is hypoplastic; the left vertebral artery is the main artery contributing to the basilar artery.

may still wish to undergo surgery, particularly if they experience recurrent TIAs. In the re-analysis of the European Carotid Surgery Trial, endarterectomy did reduce the risk of recurrent TIA in patients with near occlusion. However, patients should be informed that endarterectomy does not prevent stroke.

The trials do not address the issue of treatment in cases such as the current one in which it can be difficult to determine the source of the emboli and whether endarterectomy is beneficial in cases where emboli from one carotid artery travel to the contralateral hemisphere owing to aberrant flow. In such cases, decisions must be made on an individual patient basis after discussion between physicians, surgeons, and the patient.

In this patient, endarterectomy would not just have reduced the risk of further embolization, but would probably also have improved overall blood flow to the brain, given his contralateral occlusion. This is particularly the case for patients with severe posterior circulation stenoses. Since surgical risk is higher in patients with contralateral occlusion, such patients may also be considered for carotid stenting (see Case 19).

Further reading

Rothwell PM, Warlow CP on behalf of the European Carotid Surgery Trialists' Collaborative Group (2000). Low risk of ischemic stroke in patients with reduced internal carotid artery lumen diameter distal to severe symptomatic carotidstenosis: cerebral protection due to low poststenotic flow. *Stroke*; **31**: 622–30.

Rothwell PM, Eliasziw M, Gutnikov SA, *et al.*, on behalf of the Carotid Endarterectomy Trialists' Collaboration (2003). Analysis of pooled data from the randomised controlled trials of endarterectomy for symptomatic carotid stenosis. *Lancet*; **361**: 107–16.

Rothwell PM, Gutnikov SA, Warlow CP, on behalf of the European Carotid Surgery Trialist's Collaboration (2003). Reanalysis of the final results of the European Carotid Surgery Trial. *Stroke*; **34**: 514–23.

Case 11

A 22-year-old woman presented to her GP with a 3-day history of acute-onset rotational vertigo and blurred vision. Her symptoms had already improved, although she continued to feel a bit 'woozy' and unsteady. She was diagnosed with labyrinthitis. Six weeks later she was admitted to hospital after suddenly developing unsteadiness, nausea, blurred vision, and clumsiness of her right hand.

The patient had a background of systemic lupus erythematosus (SLE) and had developed nephrotic syndrome 6 months earlier. This resolved after treatment with mycophenolate and prednisolone, and renal function was normal at the time of admission. The patient continued on mycophenolate and reducing-dose steroids (currently prednisolone 15mg). She had also had an episode of herpes zoster, affecting the right mandibular nerve, approximately 3 months earlier. This resolved after treatment with oral aciclovir. She did not smoke, was not diabetic, had normal blood pressure, and there was no family history of stroke.

Questions

1. Figure 11.1 shows the patient's MRI brain scan. Describe the abnormal findings.

2. Figure 11.2 shows the patient's cerebral angiogram. Describe the angiographic appearance. From the history, what are the two most likely causes for this appearance?

3. How would you differentiate between the two causes? Which further investigations would you do to support your diagnosis?

4. Which risk factor for developing this particular vasculopathy does the patient have? How does the presentation of this vasculopathy differ from patients without this risk factor?

5. How would you treat this patient?

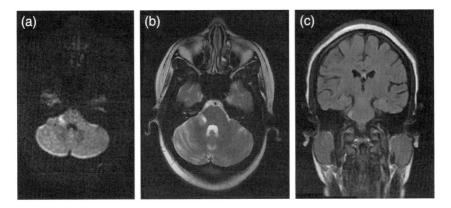

Fig. 11.1 DWI (a), axial T2-weighted image (b), and coronal FLAIR image (c).

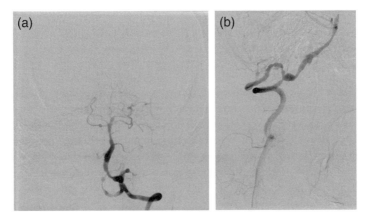

Fig. 11.2 Intra-arterial cerebral angiogram, (a) AP view and (b) lateral view of left vertebral artery injection.

Answers

1. Figure 11.1 shows the patient's MRI brain scan. Describe the abnormal findings.

The DWI (a) shows restricted diffusion in the right middle cerebellar peduncle consistent with recent ischaemic damage. This infarct is also visible in the axial T2-weighted image (b) and the coronal FLAIR image (c).

2. Figure 11.2 shows the patient's cerebral angiogram. Describe the angiographic appearance. From the history, what are the two most likely causes for this appearance?

The angiogram shows 'beading' in multiple intracranial vessels of the posterior circulation. There is narrowing in the distal left vertebral artery, the left posterior inferior cerebellar artery, the right anterior inferior cerebellar artery, and the superior cerebellar artery. Overall, the appearances are in keeping with cerebral vasculitis with involvement of large to medium size vessels. In this patient, cerebral vasculitis could be associated with her SLE. Alternatively, the varicella zoster virus (VZV) infection 4 months earlier may have caused a zoster vasculopathy.

3. How would you differentiate between the two causes? Which further investigations would you do to support your diagnosis?

The angiographic appearance is helpful in differentiating the likely cause of this patient's vasculitis. VZV vasculitis typically affects large intracranial vessels, such as the M1 segment of the MCA or, in the posterior circulation, the intracranial vertebral arteries, the basilar artery, and the P1 segments of the posterior cerebral artery, as in our patient. The vasculopathy associated with SLE typically affects small vessels. However, this distinction is by no means absolute. A recent review suggested that both small and large vessels are frequently involved in zoster vasculitis, and large vessel involvement has also been described in SLE. In our patient, the angiographic appearance is in keeping with the typical picture of VZV vasculitis.

To confirm a diagnosis of VZV vasculitis, in addition to the history of recent zoster infection and the angiographic appearance, CSF examination may be helpful. In both SLE and VZV vasculitis, this may be normal or show mild inflammatory changes with lymphocytic pleocytosis and raised protein, but usually normal glucose levels. In suspected VZV vasculitis, the CSF should also be examined for VZV-PCR and antibodies to VZV. While the PCR may often be negative, there is usually intrathecal production of immunoglobin G (IgG) antibody to VZV. Some authors suggest that for a firm diagnosis of VZV vasculopathy, CSF should be positive for either VZV-DNA or intrathecal IgG-antibodies to VZV.

Zoster vasculitis is thought to be due to direct viral infection of the cerebral blood vessels and the associated inflammatory response. It is not thought to be due to a secondary autoimmune response with cross-reactivity between viral and auto-antigens. Histopathological studies have shown viral inclusion bodies as a sign of direct viral infection in patients with VZV vasculopathy. The condition is a relatively common cause of stroke in children, but its exact incidence in adults is uncertain. It occurs more frequently in immunocompromised individuals. About half of immunocompromised patients and 16% of immunocompetent patients report a zoster rash prior to developing vascular symptoms, which can be helpful in making the diagnosis. However, there is often a delay of several weeks or months between the rash and the vascular symptoms, and often no rash is reported at all; therefore the diagnosis of VZV vasculitis should also be considered in individuals without a history of recent zoster infection or reactivation. In addition to the history, MRI brain is helpful in that it will usually be abnormal and show large vessel infarctions or scattered smaller infarcts at the border between grey and white matter. Vascular imaging and viral studies are also required to make the diagnosis. There should be evidence of viral DNA or antiviral IgG in the CSF, and usually the patient will have ischaemic changes on MRI and vasculitic changes on MRA. A definite diagnosis would require showing viral invasion of the vessel walls, but that is clearly not practical.

4. Which risk factor for developing this particular vasculopathy does the patient have? How does the presentation of this vasculopathy differ from patients without this risk factor?

Our patient is on immunosuppressive treatment for her lupus nephropathy. Immunocompromised patients are more prone than immunocompetent individuals to developing zoster vasculopathy, and they are at risk for developing more widespread disease. For example, while in immunocompetent patients often only the large intracranial vessels are affected by the virus, in immunocompromised patients there is a higher risk of small vessels and even brain tissue also being affected. Therefore immunocompromised patients may require prolonged antiviral therapy to treat a more extensive infection.

A potential complication when treating our patient is her history of renal disease. Aciclovir can cause renal impairment, in particular in patients with a pre-existing nephropathy and if it is given intravenously. Therefore the patient's renal function will have to be monitored closely during treatment, and the aciclovir dose may have to be adjusted accordingly.

5. How would you treat this patient?

VZV vasculopathy is due to active viral infection of blood vessels. Therefore treatment should consist of antiviral treatment, usually with intravenous aciclovir. However, no trial data are available, and the most effective dose and duration of treatment are currently unknown. Generally, a dose of 10–15mg/kg body weight three times daily is given for a duration of at least 14 days, although different case series report treatment durations between 10 and 28 days. As the infection usually also causes an inflammatory response, some authors recommend giving steroids concurrently with the antiviral treatment. One suggested dose is 1mg/kg bodyweight for 5 days. It is uncertain if this improves outcome. Longer immuno-suppression should probably be avoided to prevent further viral replication. Treatment response can be monitored by observing if the patient develops any new symptoms, and by repeated CSF studies for a persisting inflammatory response and viral antibodies. If there is evidence of persisting disease activity, especially in immunocompromised patients, some authors recommend continuing oral treatment with valaciclovir for 1–2 months.

Further reading

Gilden D, Cohrs RJ, Mahalingam R, Nagel MA (2009). Varicella zoster virus vasculopathies: diverse clinical manifestations, laboratory features, pathogenesis, and treatment. *Lancet Neurology*; **8**: 731–40.

Küker W (2007). Cerebral vasculitis: imaging signs revisited. *Neuroradiology*; **49**: 471–9.

Case 12

A 43-year-old nurse described episodes of multiple left hemisensory problems. She originally noticed left leg numbness, 'as if frozen', which came on suddenly after standing. This lasted for 10 minutes and then spontaneously improved. Over the next few days, she had similar episodes of left and sometimes right leg numbness, accompanied by a blurred patch in the upper nasal field of her right eye. She also experienced fleeting numbness and weakness in her left thumb and left-sided facial numbness. She had been slightly clumsy doing up buttons. She had no history of migraine, cardiac disease, or vascular disease, and was a non-smoker. She had always been an anxious character, but felt that this had worsened over the past few months.

On examination her blood pressure was 130/80mmHg and her heart rate was 68bpm, with normal respiratory and cardiovascular examinations and no carotid bruits. Neurological and fundoscopy examinations were unremarkable. Her blood results and CT head were entirely normal.

Question—Part 1

1. What do you think is the most likely diagnosis and why?

Answer

1. What do you think is the most likely diagnosis and why?

This woman presented with multiple brief episodes of sensory disturbance, affecting different parts of her body. The distribution of the sensory symptoms is in a non-anatomical distribution; it does not suggest involvement of a particular nerve, nerve root, the spinal cord, or part of the brain. There is also a vague description of visual blurring, and while she describes clumsiness, there is no evidence of this on examination. The temporal pattern of sudden onset and duration could be in keeping with transient ischaemia but, given the different locations, this would require involvement of multiple vascular territories. While focal seizures might produce transient sensory symptoms (see Case 23), these would usually be due to an underlying focal lesion and therefore would not affect multiple changing locations. The episodes sound too short-lived to be due to an underlying inflammatory process. A space-occupying lesion in the nervous system should also usually cause more permanent symptoms and, unless multifocal, should only cause symptoms in the dependent part of the body. A further possible diagnosis is migraine, although the attacks again appear to be too short-lived and the patient at no point appears to have had an associated headache. While not impossible, this appears an unlikely diagnosis. Given the non-anatomical distribution of symptoms and the normal examination, a functional non-organic aetiology is also possible. In a young woman with 'odd' symptoms, an underlying autoimmune disorder, such as lupus (see Case 25) or vasculitis (see Case 11), and multiple sclerosis (see Case 13) also have to be considered, although her symptoms appear too short-lived for these. Furthermore, there were no features in her history suggestive of an autoimmune disorder, nor were there any systemic manifestations of such a condition on examination. At this stage, the patient was diagnosed as having functional non-organic symptoms.

The patient attended the emergency department 3 weeks later with sudden-onset left-sided weakness and sensory loss predominantly affecting her face and arm, as well as slight dysarthria. Physical examination revealed left facial and arm weakness, reduced perception of pinprick over the left arm, the left side of the trunk, and the face, and mild dysarthria.

Questions—Part 2

2. What do you now think is the most likely diagnosis?

3. The patient's MRI and MRA scans are shown in Fig. 12.1. What is the diagnosis, and how would you investigate this patient further?

4. Comment on the clinical differentiation between 'organic' and 'non-organic' neurological disease.

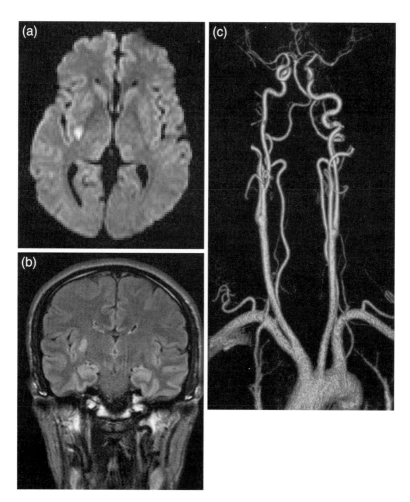

Fig. 12.1 (a) DWI, (b) coronal FLAIR of the brain, and (c) MRA of the brain-supplying arteries.

Answers

2. What do you now think is the most likely diagnosis?

The patient's symptoms and signs are now in keeping with a right subcortical lesion, i.e. they are in an 'anatomical' distribution which is much more suggestive of an organic lesion. The sudden onset suggests a vascular aetiology, and the most likely diagnosis is an ischaemic or, less likely, haemorrhagic event affecting the right MCA territory or possibly the brainstem.

3. The patient's MRI and MRA scans are shown in Fig 12.1. What is the diagnosis, and how would you investigate this patient further?

The MRI shows an acute infarct in the right lentiform nucleus; otherwise there is no abnormality, and the MRA is normal. The patient is young and has no vascular risk factors. It is unlikely that her stroke is due to atheromatous disease, and she requires investigations for more unusual causes. While her MRI only shows an isolated lesion, it is possible that some of her previous symptoms were due to ischaemia, and that she has had multiple ischaemic events. She should be investigated with transthoracic and transoesophageal echocardiography for possible sources of cardioembolism, such as endocarditis, valvular lesions, intracardiac thrombus, or a myxoma, and bubble testing to look for a PFO (see Cases 4, 37, 47, and 48). ECG and Holter monitoring should be done to look for paroxysmal arrhythmias (see Case 22).

Cervical artery dissections or vasculitis should be considered (see Cases 11, 24, and 25). However, the patient's normal MRA makes this unlikely, although separate and more detailed imaging of the intracranial vessels should also be done. If there is any diagnostic uncertainty, it may be advisable to proceed to formal intra-arterial angiography. Blood tests should be done to look for systemic inflammation, auto-antibodies pointing towards a vasculitis, and an underlying thrombophilia. If a vasculitis is suspected, examination of the CSF may also be helpful if it shows inflammatory changes. In addition to all these investigations, standard vascular risk factors for early atheroma, such as smoking history, diabetes, hypertension, and family history of vascular disease, also have to be assessed, although none of these were present in the current patient. Her blood tests revealed hyperthyroidism and a 5-day R-test showed brief episodes of AF, but echocardiography was normal. A diagnosis of cardioembolism due to paroxysmal atrial fibrillation (PAF) secondary to thyrotoxicosis was made. The patient was anticoagulated while her hyperthyroidism was treated. Her anxiety and intermittent neurological symptoms settled over the next few months.

4. Comment on the clinical differentiation between 'organic' and 'non-organic' neurological disease.

This patient was initially diagnosed as having non-organic functional symptoms, but later re-attended hospital with a stroke. In retrospect it appears likely that at least some of her previous symptoms were also ischaemic in origin, although given the wide range of symptoms, there may still have been a degree of exaggeration. As this case shows, it can be very difficult to differentiate between 'organic' and 'non-organic' symptoms. This is a highly debated issue, with discussions even concerning the terminology of 'functional', 'non-organic', or 'psychogenic', and the field is too extensive to cover in detail (see Case 20 for further discussion). However, there may be some markers to diagnose one or the other.

The patient gave a history of multiple symptoms in varying locations. Multiplicity of symptoms, often also affecting other body systems, is frequently found in patients with non-organic symptoms. Other markers of 'non-organicity' are symptom distribution in a non-organic pattern and a large number of previous attacks. Signs on examination which support a diagnosis of functional disease include a drift without pronation when checking for pronator drift, Hoover's sign (no strength on hip extension when testing this directly, but strong hip extension when testing contralateral hip flexion), or sensory loss in a non-anatomical distribution, especially when it is respecting external boundaries, such as a unilateral glove-like distribution to the elbow, or strictly the midline of the body. None of these is entirely foolproof, and further investigations will usually be requested if there is a degree of uncertainty. Again, this is open to debate, as one of the mainstays of managing patients with multiple presumed functional symptoms is to avoid over-investigation.

A recent review of neurology outpatients found that approximately 4% of patients with a diagnosis of 'conversion disorder' will later be diagnosed with organic disease. The authors point out the value of a positive diagnosis of conversion symptoms, and suggest that the fear of missing disease may be too high, as the misdiagnosis rate is low. This was further supported by a recent review which found that in only 0.4% of patients diagnosed with non-organic symptoms was the diagnosis later changed to a neurological disease that explained the patient's symptoms. The patient described here has to be seen in this context. Nevertheless, the case also stresses the importance of keeping an open mind once a diagnosis of non-organic disease is made, as sometimes only progression over time will give the diagnosis. Furthermore, not infrequently organic and non-organic symptoms may present simultaneously, which will make it more difficult to reach a definite diagnosis.

Further reading

Stone J (2009). The bare essentials: functional symptoms in neurology. *Pract Neurol*; **9**: 179–89.

Stone J, Smyth R, Carson A, *et al.* (2005). Systematic review of misdiagnosis of conversion symptoms and 'hysteria'. *BMJ*; **331**: 989.

Case 13

A 24-year-old man was referred to the rapid access TIA clinic with multiple episodes of odd sensations in the left arm and leg associated with a feeling of weakness in the left arm that had occurred over the previous 4 weeks. The first episode was preceded by a peculiar sensation in his head and he felt that things were 'moving around him'. The symptoms lasted for a few seconds before resolving completely. On a couple of occasions, he had had several episodes in a single day. He denied any nausea, double vision, or speech disturbance, and was otherwise well. He had a past history of mild hypercholesterolaemia but nothing else. General and neurological examination, including fundoscopy, was unremarkable. He had seen a private neurologist at the start of the illness who thought he might have had a stroke.

Investigations showed the following:

◆ Bloods: unremarkable

◆ Transthoracic echocardiography (TTE) (done privately): normal study.

◆ MRI brain and contrast-enhanced MRA of the cervical and intracranial vessels are shown in Fig. 13.1.

Questions

1. Give a differential diagnosis for this man's symptoms.
2. What does the MRI scan show?
3. What is the most likely diagnosis?
4. What other investigations would you request?

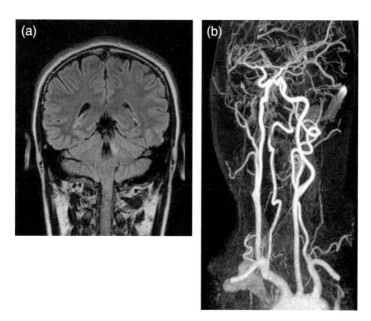

Fig. 13.1 MRI brain (a, coronal FLAIR image) and CE-MRA (b).

Answers

1. Give a differential diagnosis for this man's symptoms.

This man has multiple very transient symptoms affecting his left arm and leg. This history is not consistent with cerebral ischaemia. Recurrent ischaemia in a given vascular territory can cause repeated stereotyped symptoms, for example with MCA stenosis or in low-flow TIA (see Case 38). However, the very brief duration of symptoms makes this unlikely. Stereotyped sensory symptoms raise the possibility of seizures (see Case 23), although the symptoms appear to be too brief to be consistent with this diagnosis. Demyelination should be considered in a young person with focal neurological symptoms. Although this patient had no past history of neurological problems, this could be his first symptomatic episode.

2. What does the MRI scan show?

The coronal FLAIR image shows an area of high signal in the left middle cerebellar peduncle (arrow, Fig 13.2). On further imaging (not available) this was not associated with restricted diffusion, but there was a small area of contrast-enhancement within the lesion. Possible causes for this appearance include stroke and an inflammatory process.

The MRA of the carotid and vertebral arteries shows an unusual appearance in the V3 portion of the right vertebral artery with an apparent short segment stenosis (Fig. 13.3), but the source images were more suggestive of an image reconstruction artefact as a cause of this appearance. However, a focal vertebral artery dissection cannot be completely excluded. The extra- and intracranial vessels appear otherwise normal.

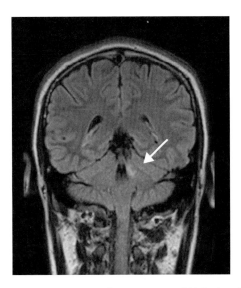

Fig. 13.2 Coronal MRI FLAIR. The arrow shows an area of high signal in the left cerebellar peduncle.

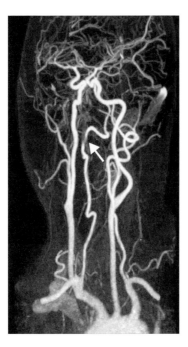

Fig. 13.3 MRA shows a possible filling defect in the distal right vertebral artery (arrow). This turned out to be an artefact rather than a genuine stenosis.

The small white matter hyperintensity in the left middle cerebellar peduncle has a relatively wide differential diagnosis including ischaemic and demyelinating aetiologies. The normal DWI sequence excludes acute ischaemia. A CTA examination could be considered to evaluate further the equivocal findings in the right vertebral artery.

3. What is the most likely diagnosis?

The most likely diagnosis was felt to be demyelination.

The MRA findings were felt to be artefactual, and even if a dissection of the right vertebral artery had occurred, this would not have caused a left cerebellar preduncle infarct. There was no history of head or neck trauma, and although the patient had mildly elevated cholesterol there were no other risk factors and no signs of a systemic disorder. In view of the transient stereotyped nature of his symptoms and the MRI findings, demyelination was felt to be most likely.

4. What other investigations would you request?

Further investigations include CSF examination and evoked potentials. This man was admitted as a day case for further investigation. CSF examination showed the presence of oligoclonal bands with a protein of 472mg/L and four lymphocytes. Evoked potentials were normal.

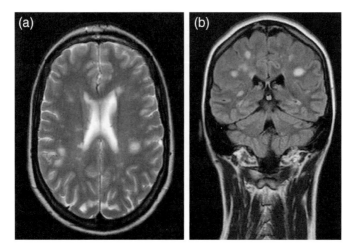

Fig. 13.4 Typical imaging appearance of multiple sclerosis. The axial T2 (a) and coronal FLAIR (b) images show multiple ovoid lesions in the subcortical and periventricular white matter. Typically, lesions are also found in infratentorial regions—not shown here.

The patient's symptoms resolved after some months. The final diagnosis was of a demyelinating event. He was concerned about multiple sclerosis. Multiple sclerosis (MS) is a common chronic disorder of the CNS, characterized pathologically by areas of inflammatory demyelination that spread throughout the CNS over time. Although the clinical course is highly variable, most patients eventually develop severe neurological disability. In 85% of patients who later develop MS, clinical onset is with an acute or subacute episode of neurological disturbance due to a single white matter lesion. This presentation is known as a 'clinically isolated syndrome'. Around 21% of those with a clinically isolated syndrome present with optic neuritis, 46% with long-tract symptoms and signs, 10% with a brainstem syndrome, and 23% with multifocal abnormalities. The presentation of MS affects disease course and prognosis, with sensory symptoms having a good prognosis. The presence and number of lesions on MRI also affects prognosis, with the risk of a diagnosis-defining second episode being higher in those with an abnormal scan and increasing with the number of lesions seen (see Fig. 13.4) and also in those with CSF abnormalities.

The patient was informed that a diagnosis of multiple sclerosis could not be made on the basis of an isolated episode of demyelination. His risk of developing MS would probably be considered low to intermediate in view of the clinical presentation, single lesion on scan, and abnormal CSF.

Further reading

Bourdette D, Simon J (2009). The radiologically isolated syndrome: is it very early multiple sclerosis? *Neurology*; **72**: 780–1.

Fazzone HE, Lefton DR, Kupersmith MJ (2003). Acute occipital demyelinating lesion appearing as an infarct on diffusion magnetic resonance imaging. *Am J Ophthalmol*; **135**: 96–7.

Miller, D, Barkhof, F, Montalban, X, *et al.* (2005). Clinically isolated syndromes suggestive of multiple sclerosis, part I: natural history, pathogenesis, diagnosis, and prognosis. *Lancet Neurol*; **4**: 281–8.

Okuda, DT, Mowry, EM, Beheshtian A, *et al.* (2009). Incidental MRI anomalies suggestive of multiple sclerosis: the radiologically isolated syndrome. *Neurology*; **72**: 800–5.

O'Riordan S, Nor AM, Hutchinson M (2002). CADASIL imitating multiple sclerosis: the importance of MRI markers. *Mult Scler*; **8**: 430–2.

Reidel MA, Stippich C, Heiland S, Storch-Hagenlocher B, Jansen O, Hähnel S. (2003). Differentiation of multiple sclerosis plaques, subacute cerebral ischaemic infarcts, focal vasogenic oedema and lesions of subcortical arteriosclerotic encephalopathy using magnetisation transfer measurements. *Neuroradiology*; **45**: 289–94.

Zivadinov R, Bergsland N, Stosic M, *et al.* (2008). Use of perfusion- and diffusion-weighted imaging in differential diagnosis of acute and chronic ischemic stroke and multiple sclerosis. *Neurol Res*; **30**: 816–26.

Case 14

A 50-year-old man developed sudden-onset vertigo, headache, vomiting, and poor balance. He was admitted to hospital. On the next day, he developed slurred speech, photophobia, and a stiff neck and became increasingly drowsy. His temperature was 38.5°C, blood pressure 190/100mmHg, and heart rate 110bpm. His Glasgow Coma Scale (GCS) was recorded as 11, and he was sedated and intubated.

There was no past medical history of note, and no history of recent infection or foreign travel. There were no vascular risk factors apart from moderate obesity (body mass index (BMI) 29).

Questions

1. What is the differential diagnosis?
2. The patient's CT scans on arrival and on the following day are shown in Figs 14.1 and 14.2. Describe the findings, and compare the figures. Which complication has developed?
3. How would you manage this patient further?

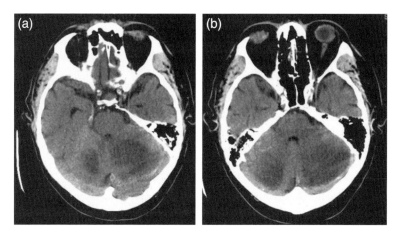

Fig. 14.1 CT brain scan on arrival in hospital.

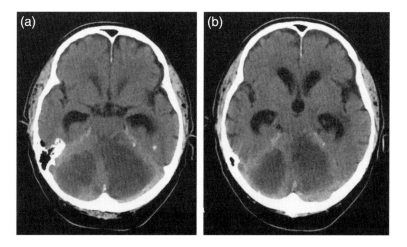

Fig. 14.2 CT brain scan one day later.

Answers

1. What is the differential diagnosis?

The sudden onset of symptoms suggests that this patient has had a vascular event. Given his symptoms of vertigo, poor balance, and headache, it is likely that the posterior circulation is affected. The original symptoms are entirely in keeping with a brainstem or cerebellar stroke.

The raised temperature and gradually decreasing level of consciousness over the next day might indicate an infection, for example encephalitis. However, the original symptom onset was sudden, with no prodrome. This makes an underlying infection or inflammatory process less likely. Similarly, a systemic vasculitis causing a stroke would be unusual in the absence of any preceding symptoms. It is much more likely that the deterioration is a consequence of the stroke rather than an aetiological feature.

A decreased level of consciousness may be a sign of increased intracranial pressure, as may hypertension and a raised temperature (neurogenic fever). A possible complication of a cerebellar stroke is the development of hydrocephalus, with subsequent increased intracranial pressure and brainstem compression. This occurs particularly in young patients, who do not usually have any brain atrophy. It is the most likely diagnosis in this patient.

2. The patient's CT scans on arrival and on the following day are shown in Figs 14.1 and 14.2. Describe the findings, and compare the figures. Which complication has developed?

The CT brain scan shows bilateral cerebellar infarcts. On the first scan, which was done one day after symptom onset, the fourth ventricle and basal cisterns are patent. The second CT scan was done one day later, after the patient had become increasingly drowsy. It shows swelling of the infarcts, compression of the fourth ventricle, and obliteration of the basal cisterns. As CSF outflow is obstructed by the compressed fourth ventricle, acute hydrocephalus has developed, and the temporal horns of the lateral ventricles are dilated.

3. How would you manage this patient further?

This patient's intracranial pressure may increase further and lead to rapid deterioration and death. Given that the patient is young and was previously healthy, and that the original neurological deficit appears to have been relatively mild, his chances of recovery from the original stroke should be good if his hydrocephalus is treated. He should be transferred to a neurosurgical unit immediately.

Possible neurosurgical interventions include insertion of an extraventricular drain (EVD) to drain CSF from the lateral ventricles. While straightforward, this induces the risk of upward herniation of the brainstem. A further intervention is posterior fossa decompression. This consists of removal of bone from the posterior fossa, which allows the swollen cerebellum to expand outside the posterior fossa without further brainstem compression. Some authors also recommend additional

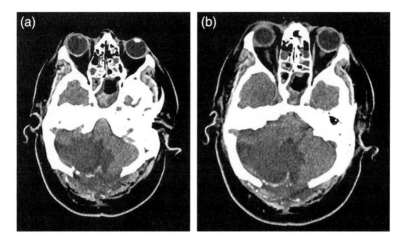

Fig. 14.3 CT brain scan after posterior fossa decompression. The scan shows the established infarct in the right and medial parts of the left cerebellar hemisphere. There is a large bony defect in the occipital skull bone.

removal of the infarcted cerebellar tissue. There is still some debate about which patients are most likely to benefit from surgery, the timing of surgery, and which surgical method should be used in which patients. However, overall there is much less debate about the indication and benefit of decompressive surgery after a cerebellar stroke than after a large hemispheric stroke (see Case 24). The American and European guidelines for acute stroke management recommend surgical intervention to relieve hydrocephalus and brainstem compression in patients with large cerebellar strokes.

After the neurosurgical intervention, the patient should be investigated for the cause of his stroke. This should include imaging of the posterior circulation vessels to look for a vertebral artery dissection, a common cause of stroke in younger patients, or early atheromatous disease. Cardiac investigations to look for a cardioembolic source as well as blood tests for diabetes, hypercholesterolaemia, autoimmune disease, and a possible thrombophilia should also be done and secondary preventative treatment started as appropriate.

The patient continued to deteriorate rapidly. Although he was treated with an EVD and posterior fossa decompression, this was probably done too late. He did not recover and died some days later. Figure 14.3 shows the CT scan of another patient after a posterior fossa decompression for a right-sided cerebellar infarct. The extensive bony defect is clearly visible. This patient eventually made a good recovery.

Key point

Hydrocephalus after a cerebellar stroke, whether ischaemic or haemorrhagic, is a common complication, in particular in young people without cerebellar atrophy, who have less intracranial 'space' which would allow the brain to swell. The typical presentation is that of a patient with a posterior circulation event who subsequently develops a deteriorating level of consciousness and further brainstem signs in addition to those caused by the initial event. Cerebellar swelling will usually be at its maximum 2–4 days after the stroke, but may occur on the same day or up to 9 days later. Patients with large cerebellar strokes should be observed closely for changes in their level of consciousness and new neurological signs. The threshold for re-scanning to check for hydrocephalus should be low. Similarly, patients with hydrocephalus and no contraindications to surgery should be discussed with the neurosurgeon at an early stage to consider neurosurgical intervention.

Further reading

Adams HP, Jr, del Zoppo G, Alberts MJ, *et al.* (2007). Guidelines for the early management of adults with ischemic stroke: a guideline from the American Heart Association/American Stroke Association Stroke Council. *Stroke*; **38**: 1655–1711.

Jauss M, Krieger D, Hornig C, *et al.* (1999). Surgical and medical management of patients with massive cerebellar infarctions: results of the German–Austrian Cerebellar Infarction Study. *J Neurol*; **246**, 257–64.

Jüttler E, Schweickert S, Ringleb PA, *et al.* (2009). Long-term outcome after surgical treatment for space-occupying cerebellar infarction: experience in 56 patients. *Stroke*; **40**: 3060–6.

Case 15

A 65-year-old woman was referred to the TIA clinic from the rheumatology service with an episode of right upper limb weakness. One week earlier she had stood up to turn off the television whereupon her right arm had moved across her body and begun to shake. This was associated with a difficulty expressing herself, although she was able to understand her husband. She was helped to a chair by her husband and the right arm shaking resolved immediately although the speech did not return to normal for about an hour. On direct questioning, she admitted three similar but more minor episodes that had all occurred when standing but had resolved shortly after sitting down. The first episode had occurred 4 months earlier.

There was a past history of hypertension and psoriasis, and she was taking candesartan. Six months earlier she had been diagnosed with giant cell arteritis (GCA) following loss of vision in the right eye. She had been started on high-dose steroids but, despite this, her vision had continued to deteriorate and pulsed cyclophosphamide had been introduced. At the time of presentation to the TIA clinic she was in remission and had been for the last 4 months. Four weeks before being seen in the TIA clinic, she had been noted by the rheumatologists to be febrile and in AF at a rate of 110bpm. Beta-blockers and aspirin had been started and a referral to the cardiologists had been made.

Her medications were sotalol 80mg twice daily, aspirin 75mg, cyclophosphamide (cyclical), prednisolone 30mg once daily, and ramipril 5mg twice daily.

On examination, she was cushingoid, her pulse was regular at 60bpm, and her blood pressure was 120/70mmHg. There was no neurological abnormality.

Investigations done in the TIA clinic showed the following:

◆ ESR 10, CRP 4
◆ ECG: sinus rhythm.
◆ MRI and MRA are shown in Figs 15.1, 15.2, and 15.3.

Questions

1. What cerebrovascular syndrome does this case illustrate? Why might the most recent episode of focal neurological symptoms have been the worst?
2. What do the MRI and MRA scans in Figs 15.1–15.3 show? What do the arrows indicate?
3. Is the history of GCA relevant to the MRA abnormalities?
4. How would you manage this patient?

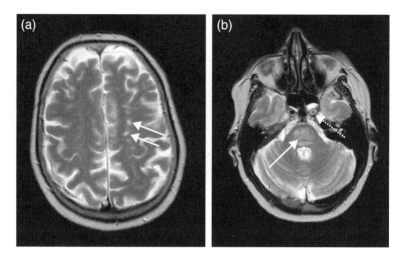

Fig. 15.1 MRI brain, axial T2-weighted images.

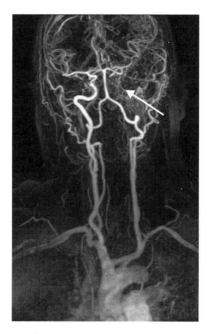

Fig. 15.2 CE-MRA of the cervical and intracranial arteries.

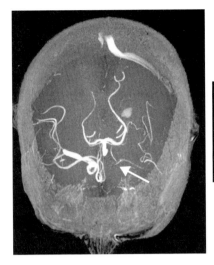

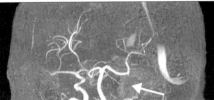

Fig. 15.3 Intracranial TOF-MRA.

Answers

1. What cerebrovascular syndrome does this case illustrate? Why might the most recent episode of focal neurological symptoms have been the worst?

This case illustrates the syndrome of limb shaking TIAs.

The patient gives a clear history of focal cerebrovascular symptoms precipitated by standing up and relieved by sitting down (after an interval). The description of the arm moving across the body followed by jerking of the arm is typical of the syndrome. The mechanism is poorly understood but is associated with poor cerebral perfusion, usually a combination of systemic low blood pressure, often induced by a postural change, and cerebrovascular stenosis (see Case 38 for further discussion). In this case, the poor perfusion must have affected the left cerebral hemisphere in view of the right-sided symptoms and speech disturbance.

According to the patient, the latest episode of limb-shaking TIA was the worst. The recent diagnosis of AF had resulted in a prescription of sotalol, a β-blocker designed to slow the heart rate and maintain sinus rhythm should spontaneous cardioversion occur. Sotalol is likely to have lowered her blood pressure and increased the likelihood of postural hypotension and thus cerebral hypoperfusion.

2. What do the MRI and MRA scans in Figs 15.1–15.3 show? What do the arrows indicate?

The MRI (Fig. 15.1) shows small areas of watershed infarction in the left hemisphere (a). It also shows extensive small vessel disease in the pons (b, solid arrow). The dashed arrow indicates the left intracranial internal carotid artery, which is occluded and has a thickened wall. Figs 15.2 and 15.3 show an absent left internal carotid artery from the carotid bifurcation (compare to contralateral appearances, where the right internal carotid artery and right middle cerebral artery are clearly visible). The appearances are consistent with left cerebral hypoperfusion due to severe vascular occlusive disease. It is of note that, despite the complete carotid occlusion, the patient has only suffered postural focal neurological symptoms. This is surprising and suggests either a gradual process of occlusion allowing the development of collaterals or that there was already a good collateral circulation in place at the time of occlusion.

3. Is the history of GCA relevant to the MRA abnormalities?

The history of GCA is probably relevant to the MRA findings.

The mechanism of the left carotid occlusion is unclear. The possibilities include cardioembolism secondary to AF, vasculitic inflammation and secondary occlusion, and, less likely, large vessel thromboembolism.

GCA, a granulomatous vasculitis of the older adult, often manifests as temporal arteritis, sometimes in association with polymyalgia rheumatica. The vasculitis may involve the aorta and its branches, resulting in myocardial infarction, stroke, aneurysm or dissection of the aorta, and lower limb arterial thrombosis. Associations have also been found between GCA and *Chlamydia pneumoniae* infection, anti-cardiolipin antibodies, and chronic inflammation, each of which is a suspected risk factor for myocardial infarction, stroke, and aortic disease.

There are several plausible mechanisms explaining the observed association between GCA and cardiovascular disease. The focal vasculitis of GCA may produce acute arterial occlusion and secondary stroke (Figs 15.4 and 15.5 show the brain imaging from another patient presenting to the TIA clinic who was found to have GCA and carotid occlusion) or myocardial infarction, or it can progress to luminal ectasia with dissection or aneurysm of the aorta. GCA may also induce reactive thrombocytosis and hyperfibrinoginaemia, predisposing to atherothrombosis. Further, there appears to be a strong dose–response relationship between markers of chronic inflammation and cardiovascular disease risk.

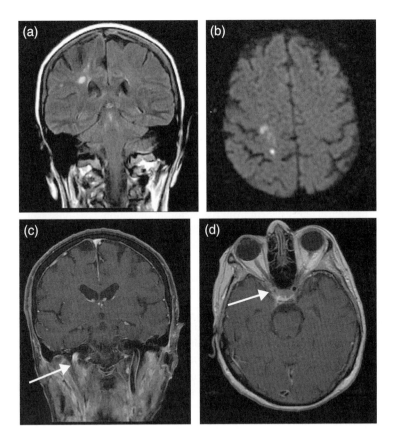

Fig. 15.4 MRI brain images from a 79-year-old woman who was referred to the TIA clinic with two episodes of transient weakness of the left hand. ESR was 121 and CRP 156 with no evidence of infection. MRI FLAIR (a) showed patchy right hemisphere deep white matter infarctions with restricted diffusion (b). Carotid doppler showed a right carotid occlusion, shown also on coronal (c) and axial (d) MRI (arrows, compare to contralateral appearance). Temporal artery biopsy confirmed giant cell arteritis. The patient required steroids and cyclophosphamide to control her disease.

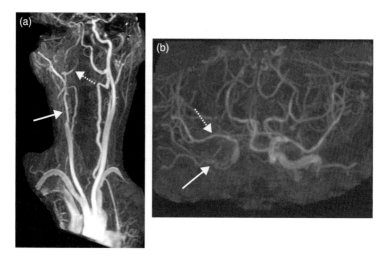

Fig. 15.5 MRA of the cervical and intracranial vessels of the patient shown in Figure 15.4. The right ICA is occluded at the level of the bifurcation (a, solid arrow) and is therefore not visible intracranially (b, solid arrow, compare to contralateral appearance). There is filling of the right middle cerebral artery via collateral branches (b, dashed arrow). The right vertebral artery is hypoplastic and terminates in the right posterior inferior cerebellar artery (a, dashed arrow).

4. How would you manage this patient?

Since patients with GCA appear to be at increased risk of cardiovascular disease, they may particularly benefit from risk factor modification. Low-dose aspirin may attenuate the inflammatory response seen with GCA, as well as the long-term risk of cardiovascular disease. Similarly, statin use may conceivably contribute to an overall reduction in cardiovascular risk among patients with GCA and increased C-reactive protein. The most likely cause of the ICA occlusion in this patient was inflammatory.

However, in view of the history of AF and her high CHADS score (see Case 22), she was switched from aspirin to warfarin. A few months later, she was admitted with a chest infection and became very confused and agitated. CT brain scan showed a small thalamic haemorrhage (Fig. 15.6). This was probably hypertensive in aetiology, although no microbleeds were seen on the GRE images (see Case 41 for discussion of microbleeds). The warfarin was stopped and aspirin was restarted after an interval. The extensive white matter changes seen on the MRI were most likely due to hypertensive small vessel disease (see Case 49).

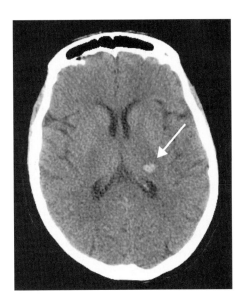

Fig. 15.6 CT brain showing a small haemorrhage in the left thalamus.

Further reading

Evans JM, O'Fallon WM, Hunder GG (1995). Increased incidence of aortic aneurysm and dissection in giant cell (temporal) arteritis: a population-based study. *Ann Intern Med*; **122**: 502–7.

Nesher G (2000). Neurologic manifestations of giant cell arteritis. *Clin Exp Rheumatol*; **18**: S24–6.

Ray JG, Mamdani MM, Geerts WH (2005). Giant cell arteritis and cardiovascular disease in older adults. *Heart*; **91**: 324–8.

Ridker PM, Rifai N, Rose L, Buring JE, Cook NR (2002). Comparison of C-reactive protein and low-density lipoprotein cholesterol levels in the prediction of first cardiovascular events. *N Engl J Med*; **347**: 1557–65

Tuhrim S, Rand JH, Wu XX, *et al.* (1999). Elevated anticardiolipin antibody titer is a stroke risk factor in a multiethnic population independent of isotype or degree of positivity. *Stroke*; **30**: 1561–5.

Van Der Meer IM, De Maat MP, Hak AE, *et al.* (2002). C-reactive protein predicts progression of atherosclerosis measured at various sites in the arterial tree: the Rotterdam Study. *Stroke*; **33**: 2750–5.

Case 16

Case 16.A

A 78-year-old right-handed woman presented with sudden-onset drowsiness and confusion. She had a vertical upgaze palsy and complained of sensory loss in the right side of her body. The patient's MRI brain is shown in Fig. 16.1.

Case 16.B

A 73-year-old woman was referred from the eye clinic where she was under glaucoma follow-up. She had noticed that when reading the newspaper, she was suddenly unable to see more than the first three letters of each word. The problem lasted for 20 minutes and persisted when she covered her eyes in turn. There was no headache or any additional neurological symptoms. She was an ex-smoker and her father had died of a myocardial infarction aged 59.

Two months later, she reported a collapse after walking down the stairs. She did not lose consciousness and had no premonitory symptoms, but for some minutes after the fall she was unable to move her arms and legs. After the weakness had resolved, her walking still felt unsteady for some hours afterwards and she felt that her vision was blurred. On examination 2 days after the event, blood pressure was 190/70mmHg and heart rate 68bpm. Cardiovascular and respiratory examinations were unremarkable. She had full visual fields, but there was mild left-sided heel–shin ataxia. ECG showed sinus arrhythmia. Echocardiography was normal and carotid ultrasound revealed an 80% stenosis of the right ICA. The patient's brain imaging is shown in Figs 16.2 and 16.3.

Questions

1. Describe the MRI findings in Fig. 16.1.
2. Which anatomical variant might explain the MRI findings?
3. In case 16.B, which visual defect is described in the first episode and which area of the brain is most likely to be involved?
4. Which vascular territory do you think is affected in the patient's second event? Do you think that the carotid stenosis is relevant to this patient's presentation?
5. Which anatomical variant explains the findings in Figs 16.2 and 16.3? How is this relevant to her clinical presentation?

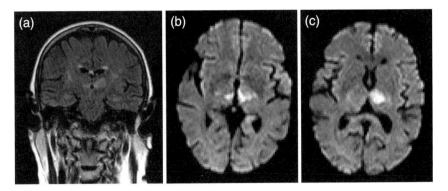

Fig. 16.1 (a) Coronal FLAIR image and (b, c) diffusion-weighted images of Case 16.A.

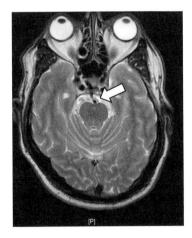

Fig. 16.2 Axial T2-weighted MRI brain, Case 16.B.

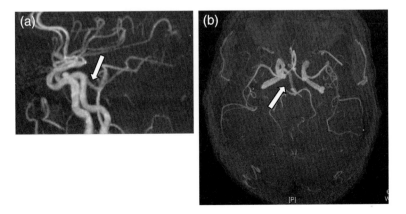

Fig. 16.3. Intracranial TOF-MRA, Case 16.B. (a) lateral view, (b) axial view.

Answers

1. Describe the MRI findings in Fig. 16.1.

The MRI scan shows bilateral thalamic infarcts, with the left one extending up to the midline and lying in the dorsum of the thalamus, and a smaller infarct on the right side. The patient has a diagnosis of bilateral thalamic infarcts.

2. Which anatomical variant might explain the MRI findings?

Simultaneous bilateral thalamic infarcts are rare and are usually due to an embolic event. They may occur as part of the 'top of the basilar syndrome', when an embolus to the top of the basilar artery may divide and embolize into both posterior cerebral arteries including the branches to the thalamus. They may also occur as a result of anatomical variants, in which part of the blood supply to both thalami arises from a unilateral blood vessel.

The blood supply to the thalamus arises from the P1 segment (between the basilar artery and the posterior communicating artery; paramedian artery) and the P2 segment (distal to posterior communicating artery; inferolateral and posterior choroidal arteries) of the posterior cerebral artery, as well as from the posterior communicating artery (tubero-thalamic arteries). While the paramedian arteries are generally bilateral, both may arise from the same unilateral P1 segment, or they may arise from a common trunk originating from one P1 segment, as shown in Fig. 16.4. This variant is called the 'artery of Percheron', and it supplies the mesial aspect of both thalami and the rostral midbrain. It occurs particularly frequently in patients with a unilateral fetal origin posterior cerebral artery, in whom the posterior cerebral artery arises from the carotid artery and the P1 segment on one side is congenitally absent. This occurs in approximately 30% of the population. Embolization into an artery of Percheron may result in occlusion of both paramedian arteries and cause bilateral thalamic infarction.

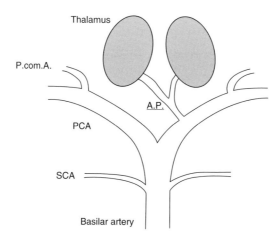

Fig. 16.4 Posterior circulation and artery of Percheron: P.com.A., posterior communicating artery; PCA, posterior cerebral artery; SCA, superior cerebellar artery; A.P., artery of Percheron.

Thalamic infarcts can present with a large variety of clinical symptoms, depending on which thalamic nuclei are affected. Infarcts in the paramedian artery territory predominantly cause deficits in arousal and memory. Left-sided infarcts may also cause speech disturbance (adynamic aphasia), whereas right-sided infarcts can result in visuospatial deficits. Bilateral infarcts can lead to severe impairment, initially with akinetic mutism or coma and at a later stage, if recovery occurs, with behavioural problems. These are often associated with eye movement abnormalities, usually due to concurrent midbrain infarction.

3. In case 16.B, which visual defect is described in the first episode and which area of the brain is most likely to be involved?

The visual field defect described is highly suggestive of a right homonymous hemianopia. A useful way to differentiate between monocular visual loss and hemianopia is to ask the patient if they covered each eye in turn. If the defect persisted with one eye covered, it is likely that the patient is describing a hemispheric field defect rather than monocular visual loss. Therefore further investigations should concentrate on looking for pathology in the visual pathway distal to and including the optic chiasm, whereas monocular visual loss should concentrate investigations on the eye and optic nerve. However, patients often find it very difficult to differentiate between a field defect and monocular visual loss (see also Case 35), and it is advisable to keep an open mind. Given the sudden onset of symptoms and the symptom duration in the patient described here, this episode of visual loss was most likely due to a TIA in the left posterior cerebral artery territory, i.e. the left occipital cortex.

4. Which vascular territory do you think is affected in the patient's second event? Do you think that the carotid stenosis is relevant to this patient's presentation?

The patient's symptoms of transient tetraparesis, gait ataxia, and possible mild double vision, which she may have perceived as blurred vision, are all highly suggestive of a posterior circulation ischaemic event, as is the examination finding of heel–shin ataxia. Given the combination of symptoms, these most likely arose from transient ischaemia in the pons, i.e. in the territory of branches from the basilar artery. In such a case, investigations should concentrate on looking for stenosis of the vertebral or basilar arteries, or other embolic sources that could cause embolization into the posterior circulation. In patients with normal cerebral vasculature, it would be highly unlikely that a carotid stenosis was related to symptoms in the brainstem. Even in the unlikely event that there was embolization through the posterior communicating artery or a fetal origin posterior cerebral artery, these emboli would cause infarction in the occipital lobes and would not reach the brainstem.

5. Which anatomical variant explains the findings in Figs 16.2 and 16.3? How is this relevant to her clinical presentation?

The patient's imaging revealed the presence of a persistent trigeminal artery (PTA) (arrows in Figs 16.2 and 16.3). This is a remnant of the fetal carotid–basilar circulation.

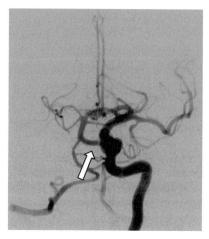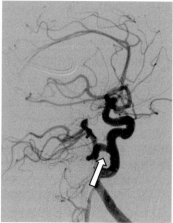

Fig. 16.5 Intra-arterial angiogram of another patient with a PTA which connects the left ICA and the basilar artery (arrows).

A PTA usually originates from the cavernous portion of the ICA and terminates in the basilar artery between the anterior inferior cerebellar artery and the superior cerebellar artery (arrows in Fig. 16.3). The angiographic prevalence of PTAs is estimated to be 0.02–1.25%. PTAs may be associated with other developmental abnormalities of the cerebral circulation, in particular with small or absent posterior communicating arteries and hypoplastic vertebral or basilar arteries. Figure 16.5 shows an angiographic example of another patient with a PTA.

PTAs may also be associated with arteriovenous malformations, aneurysms and anomalous origins of other vessels, as well as trigeminal neuralgia, subclavian steal syndrome, and Chiari malformations.

In the patient presented here, the relevance of the PTA is that it forms a connection between the carotid and the basilar arteries. Even though the patient presented with what would generally be regarded as 'posterior circulation symptoms', these may well have been caused by embolization from her carotid artery stenosis through the PTA to the basilar artery. In the absence of any other embolic source, it is very likely that this patient has a severe symptomatic carotid artery stenosis, and that she should undergo urgent carotid endarterectomy.

Further reading

Gasecki AP, Fox AJ, Lebrun LH, Daneault N (1994). Bilateral occipital infarctions associated with carotid stenosis in a patient with persistent trigeminal artery. *Stroke*; **5**: 1520–3.

Schmahmann JD (2003). Vascular syndomes of the thalamus. *Stroke*; **34**: 2264–78.

Case 17

A 29-year-old woman with a history of long-standing well-controlled type 1 diabetes mellitus presented with a one week history of horizontal double vision on looking to the left. She had noticed this after waking up one morning. In the preceding 2 weeks the patient had developed an increasingly severe generalized headache, which was particularly noticeable throughout the night and in the morning. She had vomited on several occasions, and she had also been aware of right-sided pulsatile tinnitus. Six weeks previously the patient had been treated for a presumed ear infection. Although her earache had improved, it had never quite settled. The patient denied any associated photo- or phonophobia, neck stiffness, or motor or sensory symptoms. She was feeling well within herself. Clinical examination some days after the onset of the double vision revealed a left sixth nerve palsy and bilateral papilloedema. There was no other neurological deficit.

Questions

1. What is the differential diagnosis?
2. Which investigations would you request?
3. Describe the findings in Fig. 17.1.
4. How would you treat this patient?
5. What is the prognosis of this condition?
6. How do you explain the patient's sixth nerve palsy?
7. And her tinnitus?

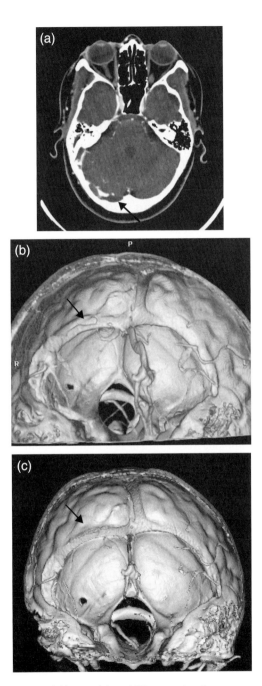

Fig. 17.1 CT venogram, axial image (a) and 3D reconstruction on presentation (b) and 6 months later (c).

Answers

1. What is the differential diagnosis?

The history in this patient suggests increased intracranial pressure, and this is further supported by her bilateral papilloedema. The close temporal relationship to the ear infection suggests that this may be an important aetiological factor. A cerebral abscess could lead to increased intracranial pressure, but we would expect the patient to be more unwell and perhaps to have additional focal signs. Transverse venous sinus thrombosis is a well-recognized complication of middle-ear infection and can lead to increased intracranial pressure. It appears likely that this is the diagnosis here.

2. Which investigations would you request?

Brain imaging and imaging of the cerebral venous system. This can be done with either a CT venogram or an MR venogram, depending on local availability and expertise.

3. Describe the findings in Fig. 17.1.

Fig. 17.1 shows the patient's CT venogram. The axial image (a) shows a filling defect in the right transverse sinus (arrow). This indicates the presence of thrombus. The 3D-reconstruction (b) confirms a filling defect in the right transverse sinus (arrow), visible as narrowing. The second 3D-image (c) was taken 6 months later and shows complete recanalization of the sinus.

4. How would you treat this patient?

In this patient, CVST is the result of an underlying infection. Therefore treatment of the infection is mandatory. The patient underwent mastoidectomy and had 6 weeks of intravenous antibiotic treatment. The best management of the CVST is perhaps more controversial. The potential benefits of anticoagulation include prevention of new thrombus formation and of other thrombotic complications (e.g. pulmonary embolism). This has to be weighed against the risks of causing intra- and extracranial haemorrhage. Only two small randomized trials totalling 79 patients have studied whether anticoagulation improves outcome. These studies were combined in a Cochrane Review, and the conclusion was 'that anticoagulant drugs are probably safe and may be beneficial for people with sinus thrombosis but results are not conclusive'. Despite this limited evidence, anticoagulation for CVST appears to be used widely, as shown in the prospective observational International Study on Cerebral Vein and Dural Sinus Thrombosis (ISCVT), in which 83% of patients were anticoagulated for a median duration of 7.7 months. Again, the duration of anticoagulation after CVST is unclear and there is not much evidence base. Extrapolating from treatment for extracranial venous thrombotic disease, the European Federation of Neurological Societies (EFNS) recommends the following durations:

◆ 3 months if CVST was secondary to a transient risk factor

◆ 6–12 months in patients with idiopathic CVST and in those with 'mild' hereditary thrombophilia

◆ indefinite anticoagulation should be considered in patients with two or more episodes of CVST and in those with one episode of CVST and 'severe' hereditary thrombophilia.

In addition to anticoagulation, thrombolysis or thrombectomy may be other treatment options for CVST, particularly in severely affected patients. However, there are no sufficient data to show that these treatments are beneficial, and they are currently not recommended. Our patient was started on full-dose low molecular weight heparin shortly after her mastoid surgery, and she then changed to warfarin, which she continued for 9 months as an interim MR venogram had shown only incomplete recanalization of her transverse sinus. Nine months after symptom onset, she had made a full recovery.

5. What is the prognosis of this condition?

The prognosis of CVST appears to be generally good. The ISCVT found that after a median follow-up of 16 months, 57% of patients had made a full recovery and a further 22% were left with minor residual symptoms. Death occurred in 8% of patients, half of which was due to the underlying condition rather than the CVST itself. The study identified the following risk factors for an unfavourable outcome: male sex, age >37 years, reduced level of consciousness, intracranial haemorrhage on admission, thrombosis of the deep cerebral venous system, CNS infection, and cancer. In this study, most of the patients were anticoagulated. Previous single-centre studies showed highly variable outcomes, with rates of death and dependency varying from 9% to 44%.

6. How do you explain the patient's sixth nerve palsy?

Sixth nerve palsy can be a 'false localizing sign' which can occur in increased intracranial pressure. There is still some controversy regarding its mechanism. The abducens nerve has a long intracranial course, and some authors propose that raised intracranial pressure may lead to stretching of the nerve with subsequent dysfunction. Alternatively, the high pressure may lead to the nerve being pressed against the petrous ligament or the ridge of the petrous bone. Finally, high intracranial pressure may lead to the brainstem being displaced backwards. As the sixth nerve emerges straight forward from the brainstem, it may be more liable to the resulting mechanical effects than other cranial nerves, which emerge more obliquely.

7. And her tinnitus?

Tinnitus is another well-recognized symptom of increased intracranial pressure. Patients often describe a pulse-synchronous 'whooshing noise' in their head. This disappears when the pressure is lowered, for example after a lumbar puncture. The mechanism of the tinnitus is thought to be turbulence created when blood flows from the hypertensive intracranial space into the low pressure of the jugular vein. This may also explain why patients can sometimes stop the sound by applying pressure to the side of the neck, presumably compressing the jugular vein.

Further reading

Einhäupl K, Bousser M-G, de Bruijn SFTM, *et al.* (2006). EFNS guideline on the treatment of cerebral venous and sinus thrombosis. *Eur J Neurol*; **13**: 553–9.

Ferro JM, Canhão P, Stam J, *et al.* (2004). Prognosis of cerebral vein and dural sinus thrombosis. Results of the International Study on Cerebral Vein and Dural Sinus Thrombosis (ISCVT). *Stroke*; **35**: 664–70.

Stam J, de Bruijn SFTM, DeVeber G (2003). Anticoagulation for cerebral sinus thrombosis (Cochrane Review). *Stroke*; **34**: 1054–5.

Case 18

A 54-year-old previously fit woman was brought to the emergency department with sudden-onset memory loss. Her husband said that they had been at home when he had told her that it was time to leave for a prearranged appointment with friends, and she appeared to have forgotten about the appointment. He went to get ready, but on his return 5 minutes later his wife was still sitting where he had left her and had no memory of the conversation they had had 5 minutes earlier. In the emergency department, she repeatedly asked why she was in hospital and had no recollection of how she had got there. She was able to remember events up until the previous week and gave accurate biographical details. Her husband said that she had been very upset by an incident of vandalism in her garden the day before presentation. She was not taking any medication and had no prior medical history. Other than the memory disturbance, examination was unremarkable.

Questions

1. What is the diagnosis? Give a differential diagnosis for this condition.
2. What are the common precipitants?
3. What is the mechanism underlying this condition?
4. How would you manage this patient?
5. What is the prognosis?

Answers

1. What is the diagnosis? Give a differential diagnosis for this condition.

The diagnosis is transient global amnesia.

TGA is a characteristic clinical syndrome that lasts for up to 24 hours. The diagnostic criteria are as follows:

- presence of an anterograde amnesia, which is witnessed by an observer
- no clouding of consciousness or loss of personal identity
- cognitive impairment limited to amnesia
- no focal neurological or epileptic signs
- no recent history of head trauma or seizures
- resolution of symptoms within 24 hours
- mild vegetative symptoms (headache, nausea, dizziness) might be present during the acute phase.

The incidence of TGA ranges from 3 to 8 per 100 000 people per year and 75% of patients are aged between 50 and 70 years. It is rare in those aged less than 40 years. TGA is characterized by a sudden onset of a memory disorder in which new memories cannot be made (anterograde amnesia) and events over the past weeks and sometimes years cannot be recalled (retrograde amnesia). The patient often asks the same questions repetitively and cannot remember what they have just done. The anterograde memory deficit is profound, but there is a milder reduction of retrograde episodic memory including executive functions and recognition. Although the core amnestic syndrome usually lasts for substantially less than 24 hours, mild subclinical neuropsychological deficits with concomitant vegetative symptoms can last for days after the episode. After resolution of symptoms the anterograde memory returns to normal, but the patient never regains memory for the period of the attack itself. There is probably also a persistent small retrograde memory loss.

The restriction of the clinical manifestations of TGA to the consequences of isolated amnesia and the lack of any other behavioural abnormality or more general confusion help to distinguish TGA from alternative diagnoses such as complex partial seizures, hypoglycaemia, etc. However, there are a small number of differential diagnoses that might occasionally clinically mimic a TGA. The body of the hippocampus is mainly supplied by the posterior cerebral artery and the head by the anterior choroidal artery branching from the internal carotidal artery. Therefore an ischaemic event in the territory of the posterior cerebral artery or the anterior choroidal artery may present with an amnestic syndrome. Similarly, strategic insults in the medial thalamus in the supply territory of the thalamo-perforate arteries can result in a diencephalic amnesia.

Transient epileptic amnesia should be considered if episodes recur and/or last for less than an hour. Hypoglycaemia or seizures related to hypoglycaemia can result in an amnestic deficit. Head trauma might result in post-traumatic amnesia, and an acute onset of herpes simplex infection or a limbic encephalitis may also cause an amnestic syndrome, although these conditions are usually accompanied by confusion and focal neurological signs, and the clinical course is usually one of deterioration. Occasionally migraine may result in temporary loss of memory. Psychogenic memory loss is uncommon. In such cases patients are able to continue acitivities of daily living as usual despite apparent loss of memory.

2. What are the common precipitants?

The known precipitants of TGA are:

◆ emotional stress

◆ sex

◆ physical stress (e.g. gardening, bathing in cold water)

◆ defecation/Valsalva manoeuvre.

Precipitating events frequently described include sudden immersion in cold or hot water, physical exertion, emotional or psychological stress, pain, medical procedures, sexual intercourse, and Valsalva-associated manoeuvres. Precipitants are reported in around 50–90% of documented attacks. In men TGA episodes occur more frequently after a strenuous physical event, whereas in women TGA is more closely associated with an emotional event, such as arousal, stress, or anxiety. In patients aged less than 56 years, TGA is associated with a past history of migraine. Certain personality traits might be relevant in the aetiology of TGA: there appears to be an increased frequency of psychological or emotional instability and a higher occurrence of a personal or family history of psychiatric disorders or phobic traits.

3. What is the mechanism underlying this condition?

The mechanism underlying TGA is unknown.

Originally TGA was thought to be a form of TIA, but case–control studies have shown no increase in vascular risk factors or risk of vascular disease in these patients. A migraine-type process has also been proposed as a cause of TGA since migraine is more common in TGA sufferers than in controls and cerebral perfusion of the medial temporal lobes has been shown to be abnormal during an attack.

Recent high-resolution imaging data suggest an involvement of memory circuits in the mesiotemporal region, as hyperintense MRI lesions can be detected in the hippocampal formation in TGA. An analysis of the functional anatomy of these lesions shows a selective distribution within the CA1 subfield of the hippocampal cornu ammonis. Further imaging findings have implicated cellular mechanisms in the development of these lesions, suggesting that the selective vulnerability of CA1 neurons to metabolic stress plays a crucial part in the pathophysiological cascade that leads to a transient perturbation of memory pathways in TGA. The presence of apparent medial temporal lobe ischaemia, as shown by DWI temporal lobe abnormality in the absence of demonstrable arterial pathology or increased risk of stroke, and the association of TGA with Valsalva manoeuvre have led to the proposal that venous congestion leading to transient ischaemia may be the cause of TGA.

4. How would you manage this patient?

Having a 'memory blank' often causes a high level of anxiety for the patient, as does witnessing an episode of TGA for any observers. Reassuring the patient and their family is the most important part of management. No investigation is necessary in isolated classical TGA, but MRI may be supportive. The aim of brain imaging in TGA is mainly to exclude other diagnoses.

In patients presenting with a classical history for TGA in the absence of previous attacks, no investigation is necessary. Patients with previous or atypical attacks should have brain imaging and electroencephalography (EEG). Strokes may cause memory loss, but the clinical features are usually different from those seen in TGA. Somnolence, gaze palsies, and corticospinal or spinothalamic tract damage suggest thalamic (dorsomedial or mamillothalamic tract) injury. Paramedian thalamic infarction, which is frequently bilateral as the arteries arise from the same stem in many people, causes particularly severe memory loss. Visual disorders such as hemianopia or upper quandrantanopia frequently accompany medial temporal lobe infarction which is probably the most frequent stroke lesion associated with memory loss.

A detailed analysis of the location of hippocampal lesions shows that almost all lesions can be selectively found in the area corresponding to the CA1 sector (Sommer sector) of the hippocampal cornu ammonis. Lesions seen on DWI can also be detected using T2-weighted images. The size of focal hyperintense lesions ranges from 1 to 5mm. Single or multiple lesions in the T2-weighted images show an oedema-like configuration and are usually clearly distinguishable from the sharply configured residual cavities of the vestigial hippocampal sulcus. Recent neuroimaging data have shown that the level of detection of hippocampal DWI lesions in patients with TGA depends on the time of imaging. The maximum level of detection occurs within 48–72 hours after the onset of symptoms, so early imaging might not detect these lesions.

5. What is the prognosis?

Recurrence rates for TGA are less than 3% per year. Thus patients can be reassured that they are most unlikely to suffer a recurrent attack.

If a patient has repetitive amnestic episodes, EEG is mandatory to exclude transient epileptic amnesia. For this reason, driving is allowed after one attack of TGA but not after repeated attacks.

Further reading

Bartsch T, Deuschl G (2010). Transient global amnesia: functional anatomy and clinical implications. *Lancet Neurol*; **9**: 205–14.

Bilo L, Meo R, Ruosi P, de Leva MF, Striano S (2009). Transient epileptic amnesia: an emerging late-onset epileptic syndrome. *Epilepsia*; **50** (Suppl 5): 58–61.

Hodges JR, Ward CD (1989). Observations during transient global amnesia: a behavioural and neuropsychological study of five cases. *Brain*; **112**: 595–620.

Hodges JR, Warlow CPW (1990). The aetiology of transient global amnesia: a case control study of 114 cases with prospective follow up. *Brain*; **113**: 639–57.

Pantoni L, Bertini E, Lamassa M, Pracucci G, Inzitari D (2005). Clinical features, risk factors, and prognosis in transient global amnesia: a follow-up study. *Eur J Neurol*; **12**: 350–6.

Case 19

Case 19.A

A 63-year-old man presented with three episodes of transient right-sided arm weakness and word-finding difficulties over the previous week. Each episode lasted 15 minutes. The patient had a history of hypertension, and had stopped smoking 5 years previously when he had a TIA, after which he had undergone endarterectomy for a left carotid artery stenosis. Carotid Dopplers showed a recurrent 80% stenosis of the left ICA.

Case 19.B

A 60-year-old woman was referred by her GP. She had a history of hypertension, but was otherwise well and usually kept very active. She had been given a private 'body check-up', which included carotid Dopplers, as a present for her 60th birthday. These were reported as showing a 70% stenosis of the right ICA. She would now like to know what to do about this stenosis.

Questions

1. How would you treat patient A?
2. What advice would you give patient B and how would you explain your recommendation?

Answers

1. How would you treat patient A?

This patient clinically has TIAs in the left MCA territory, which are very likely to originate from his high-grade left ICA stenosis. Revascularization of a recently symptomatic carotid stenosis has been shown to be highly beneficial if the degree of stenosis is 70–99%. It reduces the absolute 5-year risk of having a further ipsilateral stroke by 16%. This risk reduction is achieved by carotid endarterectomy. In recent years stenting has been proposed as a less invasive alternative to surgery. However, trial data suggest that endarterectomy is safer than stenting in the first few months after the intervention, with the risk of stroke or death being two to three times higher after stenting. Therefore carotid endarterectomy remains the procedure of choice in patients who require their first carotid artery intervention and who have no other contraindications to surgery. Carotid stenting is reserved for patients who have contraindications to surgery or in whom surgery is technically difficult, for example if they have had prior surgery or radiotherapy to the neck. Patient A has already had an endarterectomy, which will have caused scarring and will make further surgery more difficult and risky. In this case, if it is available, carotid stenting would be preferable.

Regardless of which procedure is done in this patient, it should be arranged urgently. The risk of having further events from a carotid stenosis is highest in the first few days after the original event, and is particularly high in patient A because he has already had multiple events within a short period of time. Ideally, carotid recanalization should be done within 2 weeks of symptom onset. If there is no contraindication, the patient should be started on dual antiplatelet therapy with aspirin and clopidogrel until the intervention as there is some evidence that this drug combination reduces the risk of early recurrence. Furthermore, carotid stenting will be done under dual antiplatelet cover, so the patient will already be on the correct treatment for this. Dual antiplatelet therapy will increase the risk of haemorrhage during surgery, and the best treatment regime should be discussed with the local vascular surgeons if a redo endarterectomy is considered.

2. What advice would you give patient B and how would you explain your recommendation?

This patient has an asymptomatic carotid artery stenosis. Therefore she has evidence of atheromatous disease, which should be treated appropriately, with reduction of relevant risk factors. She should receive lifestyle advice, and her blood pressure should be treated aggressively. Other risk factors (e.g. diabetes and cholesterol levels) should be checked and managed accordingly. If there is no contraindication, the patient should also be started on aspirin.

While this woman should have aggressive medical treatment of her atheromatous disease, she would probably not benefit from carotid endarterectomy. The endarterectomy trials for asymptomatic stenosis showed a marginal benefit for surgery, with an absolute annual risk reduction of 1% for preventing an ipsilateral stroke in patients with a carotid stenosis of ≥60%. However, since these studies were done, medical management for atheromatous disease has improved, and the stroke risk in asymptomatic carotid stenosis has fallen. Furthermore, the surgical risk in the endarterectomy trials was probably lower than in an everyday clinical setting. The combination of a lower risk on medical treatment and a higher 'real-life' surgical risk may well negate the benefit from surgery that was shown in the trials, particularly in women, who have a higher surgical risk than men.

Finally, all of the above obviously only applies if the results of the Doppler are reliable. One of the reasons that screening for carotid stenosis is not recommended is that it may result in false-positive scans. If there is any doubt about the reliability of the investigation result, carotid imaging should be repeated with either Doppler or MRA/CTA, which would also show the extent of any other cranio-cervical vascular stenoses. This may not change the decision for conservative management, but it would help to judge the severity of disease, guide the discussions with the patient, and inform medical treatment (e.g. how aggressively blood pressure is treated).

Further reading

Abbott AL (2009). Medical (nonsurgical) intervention alone is now best for prevention of stroke associated with asymptomatic severe carotid stenosis: results of a systematic review and analysis. *Stroke*; **40**: e573–83.

International Carotid Stenting Study Investigators (2010). Carotid artery stenting compared with endarterectomy in patients with symptomatic carotid stenosis (International Carotid Stenting Study): an interim analysis of a randomised controlled trial. *Lancet*; **375**: 985–97.

Rothwell PM, Eliasziw M, Gutnikov SA, *et al.* (2003). Analysis of pooled data from the randomised controlled trials of endarterectomy for symptomatic carotid stenosis. *Lancet*; **361**: 107–16.

Case 20

A 34-year-old right-handed man presented to the emergency department having been brought in by the police. He gave a history of having been assaulted in a pub. He had subsequently been taken to the police station where he was noted to have left-sided weakness and loss of speech. He was not able to give any history. He underwent CT brain and routine blood tests that were unremarkable. MRI brain was planned but he discharged himself.

Three days later he presented to the TIA clinic having been referred by the GP with persistent left-sided weakness and loss of speech. The history was given by his wife and through him writing down answers to questions. He was able to eat and drink, and could walk with difficulty, requiring a wheelchair for distances of more than a few metres. He was able to climb stairs. He denied neck pain. There was no history of illicit drug use but he had had depression and had self-harmed in the past. The old notes revealed several previous emergency department admissions following assault and a road traffic accident in which he sustained a right knee injury.

On examination, he looked well but was agitated at times and frustrated at being unable to speak. He was able to understand complex commands but had no spontaneous speech. He was able to name 'watch' and 'winder' after much encouragement. There was no neglect, visual fields were full, and CN examination was unremarkable. Tone in the limbs was normal, but there appeared to be severe weakness of the left arm and leg. Reflexes were symmetrical and plantars downgoing. Sensation was reduced to light touch and pinprick over the toes of the left foot.

Questions

1. What is the most likely cause of this man's symptoms and why? What other neurological symptoms and signs may commonly occur in this syndrome?

2. What other diagnoses should be excluded in a patient who sustains a focal neurological deficit after trauma?

3. Would you expect left-sided symptoms in a right-handed patient with this syndrome?

4. What is the prognosis?

Answers

1. What is the most likely cause of this man's symptoms and why? What other neurological symptoms and signs may commonly occur in this syndrome?

The most likely diagnosis is conversion disorder (DSM-IV). Conversion disorder is also known as dissociative motor disorder (ICD-10), or may be described as psychogenic, non-organic, hysterical, medically unexplained, or functional. Conversion disorder is defined in DSM-IV as 'symptoms suggesting a neurological disorder not secondary to malingering without physical cause'.

This man's symptoms and signs (speech difficulty and left-sided weakness in a right-handed individual, ability to climb stairs despite being in a wheelchair, and ability to comprehend and write without problem) cannot be explained by a single lesion in the CNS. There is also inconsistency in the findings in that speech was entirely absent and yet he was able to articulate watch and winder after much encouragement, and there was left-sided weakness without any change in reflexes or tone. The past history of depression and deliberate self-harm increase the likelihood of a conversion disorder. Symptoms commonly associated with conversion disorder are shown in Table 20.1.

Conversion disorder has been reported to affect around 9% of people with neurological symptoms, and up to 30% of those referred to neurology outpatient clinics may have medically unexplained symptoms. Conversion symptoms are currently conceptualized as physical symptoms induced by psychological trauma, conflict, or stress, although the exact mechanism is unknown. Recently, it has become clear that physical injury is also an important precipitant, as seen in the above case, and occurs in around 37% of patients with conversion disorder. Clinical features of conversion disorder associated with physical injury include younger age, weakness (versus movement disorder), paraparesis (versus hemiparesis), and neurological versus psychiatric study settings.

Functional MRI (fMRI) studies show differences in activation patterns in the primary and supplementary motor cortices in patients with conversion disorder compared with controls feigning weakness. Specifically, conversion disorder is associated with reduced and more diffuse activation of the motor cortex contralateral to the weak limb, and increased activation of basal ganglia, insula, lingual gyri, and inferior frontal cortex with hypo-activation of the middle frontal and orbitofrontal cortex.

Table 20.1 Symptoms associated with conversion disorder

Sensory	Motor
Diplopia	Paralysis
Blindness	Dysphasia
Deafness	Ataxia
Numbness	Tremor
	Seizures

In controls feigning weakness, there is activation of the contralateral supplementary motor area.

Erroneous diagnosis of conversion disorder used to be thought to be common, and it certainly appears that rates of misdiagnosis have dropped, perhaps through increased availability of brain imaging. Contemporary estimates suggest misdiagnosis rates to be low, at around 8%, and to occur most often with movement disorders, multiple sclerosis, and epilepsy, although such misdiagnosis may have serious consequences. Organic pathology is also more likely to be diagnosed as conversion disorder if symptoms appear bizarre or there is a previous psychiatric history.

2. What other diagnoses should be excluded in a patient who sustains a focal neurological deficit after trauma?

Cervical arterial dissection should be excluded.

Any patient with a history of trauma and focal neurological signs needs an urgent CT brain to exclude an acute brain lesion. However, if the CT scan appears normal, it is important not to forget that trauma may cause carotid or vertebral artery dissection and secondary brain infarction (see Case 24). If this diagnosis is suspected, the patient will require further imaging with MRI/MRA.

3. Would you expect left-sided symptoms in a right-handed patient with this syndrome?

Conversion disorder appears to affect both dominant and non-dominant sides

The symptoms in patients with conversion disorder are commonly thought to occur more often on the non-dominant side, a belief perhaps originating with psychiatrists practising psychoanalysis at the turn of the twentieth century and perpetuated more recently in several textbooks of neurology. However, three large reviews, including one from the early 1900s, have shown that symptoms seem to affect both dominant and non-dominant sides equally. Specifically, in one systematic review of the literature published since 1965, the pooled proportion of functional left-sided weakness and sensory symptoms in adults was 58% (95% confidence interval (CI) 55–61%). A much higher proportion of left-sided symptoms (66%, 95% CI 61–71%) was found in studies where laterality featured in the title of the paper. However, when laterality was not mentioned in the title, no significant difference between left and right was observed (53% on the left, 95% CI 48–57%). This difference could not be explained on the basis of sex differences between the groups or the date of the study. Functional or 'psychogenic' movement disorder was right-sided in 68% (95% CI 61–75%). Handedness did not influence symptom lateralization.

4. What is the prognosis?

The prognosis is not necessarily good despite the lack of organic pathology.

Fewer than 1% of patients referred to neurology outpatients with medically unexplained symptoms are subsequently diagnosed with an organic disease that was felt to be the cause of their original symptoms.

In the remaining vast majority of patients, the prognosis is not necessarily good despite the lack of demonstrable organic pathology. In one study, over 80% of patients with an initial diagnosis of conversion disorder still had weakness or sensory symptoms on follow-up after more than a year, and the majority of these had limitation of physical function, distress, and many other somatic symptoms. Retirement on medical grounds is common. Patients with sensory symptoms appear to do better than those with weakness. There is a high rate of psychiatric comorbidity and suicide.

Further reading

Akagi H, House A (2001). The epidemiology of hysterical conversion. In: Halligan PW, Bass C, Marshall JC (eds), *Contemporary approaches to the study of hysteria*. Oxford: Oxford University Press, pp.73–87.

Stone J, Sharpe M, Carson A, *et al.* (2002). Are functional motor and sensory symptoms really more frequent on the left? A systematic review. *J Neurol Neurosurg Psychiatry*; **73**: 578–81.

Stone J, Sharpe M, Rothwell PM, Warlow CP (2003). The 12 year prognosis of unilateral functional weakness and sensory disturbance. *J Neurol Neurosurg Psychiatry*; **74**: 591–6.

Stone J, Warlow C, Carson A, Sharpe M (2003). A 1908 systematic review of the laterality of hysterical hemiplegia. *J Neurol Neurosurg Psychiatry*; **74**: 1163–4.

Stone J, Smyth R, Carson A, *et al.* (2005). Systematic review of misdiagnosis of conversion symptoms and 'hysteria'. *BMJ*; **331**: 989.

Stone J, Carson A, Aditya H, *et al.* (2009). The role of physical injury in motor and sensory conversion symptoms: a systematic and narrative review. *J Psychosom Res*; **66**: 383–90.

Stone J, Carson A, Duncan R, *et al.* (2009). Symptoms 'unexplained by organic disease' in 1144 new neurology out-patients: how often does the diagnosis change at follow-up? *Brain*; **132**: 2878–88.

Case 21

Case 21.A

A 78-year-old woman presented to the TIA clinic with mild left-sided weakness. She was diagnosed with a right lacunar infarct. Her MRA also showed an incidental large aneurysm of the left ICA (Fig. 21.1).

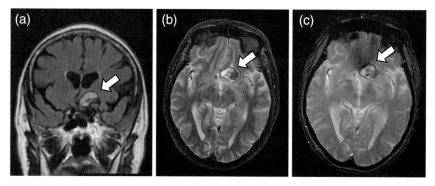

Fig. 21.1 MRI brain. Coronal FLAIR (a), axial T2-weighted (b), and GRE images (c). The arrows indicate a large aneurysm of the left ICA.

Case 21.B

A 30-year-old man presented to the neurology clinic. His mother had recently had a SAH. He had two older sisters, both of whom were well. His maternal grandmother died of a stroke at the age of 77 years. Otherwise there was no history of any vascular events in any first- or second-degree relatives. The patient was concerned that he might have inherited an aneurysm from his mother and was keen to have vascular imaging to investigate this possibility further.

Questions

1. How high do you estimate the risk of aneurysm rupture in Case 21.A? On what basis do you estimate this risk?
2. What advice would you give patient A? How would you treat her?
3. What advice would you give patient B?

Answers
1. How high do you estimate the risk of aneurysm rupture in Case 21.A? On what basis do you estimate this risk?

With the advent of non-invasive brain and cerebrovascular imaging techniques, asymptomatic intracranial aneurysms have become a relatively frequent finding. The prevalence of cerebral aneurysms in the general population is estimated to be 2–3%. However, the annual incidence of aneurysmal SAH is much lower, only about 6–9/100 000, which suggests that most aneurysms do not rupture. A number of studies of asymptomatic aneurysms have tried to identify the risk factors for aneurysm rupture. A meta-analysis of all available studies in 2007 showed that the risk of rupture increases with patient age, female gender, increasing aneurysm size, and location of the aneurysm in the posterior circulation. In addition, aneurysms were more likely to rupture if they caused symptoms (e.g. compression of a nearby structure such as the oculomotor nerve). However, compressive symptoms may simply reflect larger aneurysm size. The largest two studies to contribute to the meta-analysis were the International Study of Unruptured Intracranial Aneurysms (ISUIA), with its retrospective (ISUIA 1) and prospective (ISUIA 2) arms. These studies provided further risk estimation according to aneurysm size. Size was categorized into diameters of <7mm, 7–12mm, 13–24mm, and ≥25mm. The associated 5-year risks of rupture were as follows.

◆ Anterior circulation
  - <7mm: 0–1.5%
  - 7–12mm: 2.6%
  - 13–24mm: 14.5%
  - ≥25mm: 40%

◆ Posterior circulation
  - <7mm: 2.5–3.4%
  - 7–12mm: 14.5%
  - 13–24mm: 18.4%
  - ≥25mm: 50%

In patients with small aneurysms (<7mm), the risk of rupture was higher in patients who had previously had a ruptured aneurysm in a different location than in patients without a previous SAH. This difference was no longer present in patients with larger aneurysms.

Patient A underwent intra-arterial angiography to assess her aneurysm in detail (Fig. 21.2). The aneurysm size was measured as 22mm, giving her a 5-year risk of rupture of 14.5%, possibly higher, as the size of her aneurysm is towards the larger end of the category. Her female sex and possibly her age also put her at higher risk of rupture. However, the patient's aneurysm showed extensive calcification and thrombosis. Both of these thicken the aneurysm wall and markedly decrease the size of the lumen of the aneurysm. The calcification indicates that the aneurysm

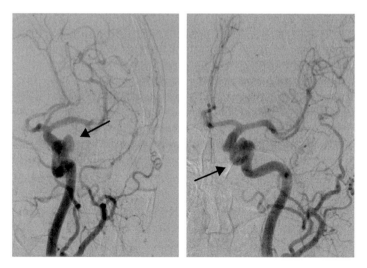

Fig. 21.2 Intra-arterial angiogram, left common carotid artery injection. The images show the aneurysm originating from the supra-ophthalmic portion of the left ICA. The aneurysm is largely thrombosed and the carotid artery is very tortuous in that region, making an intervention difficult.

may have been present for a long time without rupturing. Even though such changes have not been systematically studied, in patient A the external diameter of the aneurysm by far surpassed its lumen, and it seemed likely that this would reduce the risk of rupture.

2. What advice would you give patient A? How would you treat her?

In asymptomatic aneurysms, the risk of rupture with no intervention has to be compared with the risk of treatment. Treatment options for an aneurysm include surgical clipping and endovascular coiling. In the ISUIA studies, risk factors for a poor surgical outcome (defined as death, Rankin score 3–5, or impaired cognitive status) included increasing age, increasing aneurysm size, posterior circulation aneurysm, and previous cerebrovascular disease. In patients older than 70 years, the 1-year risk of a poor outcome was approximately 33%. Patient A had a large aneurysm and cerebrovascular ischaemia, clearly putting her into a very high surgical risk group. Endovascular coiling is the preferred treatment option in patients over the age of 50 years. However, it is also not risk free, with a 1-year risk of a poor outcome of 10–15% for patients older than 50 years with a large anterior circulation aneurysm. In addition, complete coiling of large aneurysms is often difficult to achieve, and it was felt that to a large extent spontaneous thrombosis had already achieved what would otherwise have been achieved by coiling.

Overall, this patient's risk of aneurysm rupture was probably high, although perhaps not as high as quoted in the available studies, because of the extensive thrombosis and calcification of the aneurysm. The risk of surgical intervention appeared to be unacceptably high, and endovascular intervention was also felt to be risky and to have a low chance of success as the aneurysm had a very wide opening and the vessels leading to the aneurysm were very tortuous. After reviewing all the options and discussing them with the patient, the decision was made to manage her conservatively with no intervention. She is currently doing well 1 year after her stroke and after the aneurysm was detected.

3. What advice would you give patient B?

The risk of having a cerebral aneurysm is about 2–3% in people with no family history of this condition, and the lifetime risk of having a SAH is 0.6%. In individuals who have one first-degree relative with a SAH, the risk of having an aneurysm increases to 4%, with a lifetime risk of SAH of 3.3%. The risk of having an aneurysm also depends on which first-degree relative is affected, with the risk being highest if this is a sibling. In individuals with two or more affected first-degree relatives, the risk of having an aneurysm is considerably higher at 8%, but no clear data exist regarding their lifetime risk of SAH.

Generally, screening is only recommended in individuals who have two or more first-degree relatives with a history of SAH. The chance of having an aneurysm is still low in patients with one affected first-degree relative, so that 300 at-risk people would have to be screened to avoid one fatal SAH. While screening in people with only one affected relative is therefore not effective or efficient, sometimes patients can be extremely anxious and nevertheless wish to have imaging. They should consider a number of other factors, which should be discussed with every patient before embarking on a screening programme.

- ◆ Aneurysms are not congenital but arise during life. Therefore a one-off normal vascular imaging study does not exclude the occurrence of aneurysms in the future. However, the interval at which screening should be repeated is uncertain. Intervals of 5–7 years appear reasonable. This may be done more frequently if there is a change in imaging appearances.

- ◆ If an aneurysm is found, this does not necessarily mean it should be treated. Both surgical and endovascular treatments have their risks, which may be higher than the risk of aneurysm rupture. In such a situation, some patients may find it very difficult to live with the knowledge that they have an aneurysm, even if it is small.

- ◆ Finding an aneurysm, which is then not treated, may also have implications for insurance or driving.

- ◆ Brain and vascular imaging may show up other incidental findings, which the patient may prefer not to know about, and which in themselves may raise anxiety.

- ◆ Even if the initial imaging is normal, an aneurysm may develop and rupture before the next imaging study. Screening does not offer 100% protection from SAH.

- In addition to familial SAH, patients with adult polycystic kidney disease are also at a higher risk of having cerebral aneurysms and screening should be discussed.

Patient B's personal risk of having an aneurysm and the advantages and drawbacks of screening were discussed in detail. Eventually he was happy not to be screened.

Further reading

International Study of Unruptured Intracranial Aneurysms Investigators (2003). Unruptured intracranial aneurysms: natural history, clinical outcome, and risks of surgical and endovascular treatment. *Lancet*; **362**: 103–10.

Rinkel GJE (2005). Intracranial aneurysm screening: indications and advice for practice. *Lancet Neurol*; **4**: 122–8.

Wermer MJH, van der Schaaf IC, Algra A, Rinkel GJE (2007). Risk of rupture of unruptured intracranial aneurysms in relation to patient and aneurysm characteristics: an updated meta-analysis. *Stroke*; **38**: 1404–10.

Wiebers DO, Piepgras DG, Meyer FB, *et al.* (2004). Pathogenesis, natural history, and treatment of unruptured intracranial aneurysms. *Mayo Clin Proc*; **79**: 1572–83.

Case 22

Case 22.A

An 82-year-old woman noticed that she was unable to speak properly when answering the telephone. She knew what she wanted to say and understood speech, but on speaking produced gibberish. Her symptoms persisted for 7 hours before resolving completely. There was a past history of hypertension and previous TIA 2 years previously. She was taking aspirin and amlodipine. On examination, pulse was 70bpm and regular, blood pressure was 170/80mmHg, and neurological examination was normal. Head CT revealed an old right frontal infarct. ECG confirmed sinus rhythm. Carotid Dopplers were normal.

Sixteen months later, she had a transient episode of reduced vision in the left eye that resolved. She did not seek medical attention. A week later, she was found by her niece lying in bed, not speaking, and unable to move her right side. On admission to hospital, pulse was 110bpm irregularly irregular and blood pressure was 135/90mmHg. Neurological examination showed dysphasia, gaze deviation to the left, right homonymous hemianopia, right facial palsy, and right hemiplegia.

Her ECG confirmed AF. Her CT scan showed extensive infarction in the left MCA territory (Fig. 22.1).

Case 22.B

An 84-year-old woman suddenly developed a 'drunken gait', veering to the left side when walking. These symptoms improved but did not resolve completely.

Two weeks later, while making lunch, her right hand and arm suddenly became weak and she had problems writing. She was assessed the following day at the emergency TIA clinic where she was found to have a regular pulse of 70bpm and her blood pressure was 182/106mmHg. There was reduced right handgrip. CT brain showed white matter changes and a low attenuation lesion in the anterior portion of the left corona radiata compatible with an infarct (Fig. 22.2). ECG confirmed sinus rhythm. She was discharged on aspirin, simvastatin, and an ACE inhibitor.

Eleven months later, she was admitted with left leg weakness and was discharged after a week with mild residual paresis. Investigations including repeat ECG showed nothing new.

Three years later, she had a sudden onset of right arm and leg weakness and slurred speech that came on whilst she was getting dressed. On admission to hospital, her blood pressure was 160/90mmHg and her pulse was irregular at 90bpm. There was a right facial palsy, and moderate right arm and right leg weakness. Brain CT did not show any new lesions, ECG showed AF, and carotid Doppler did not show any significant stenosis.

Questions

1. What is the likely aetiology of all the cerebral ischaemic events in the two cases outlined above?
2. Would you have managed these patients differently prior to their most recent admissions when AF was discovered?
3. What are the factors associated with increased risk of AF?
4. What secondary preventive therapy would you advise?

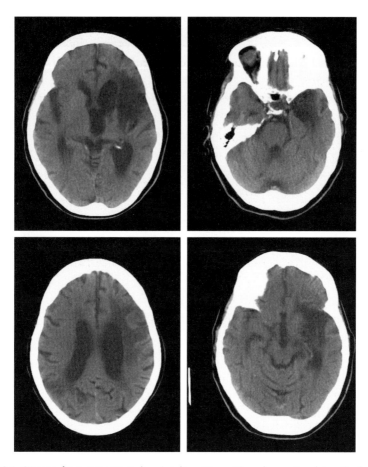

Fig. 22.1 CT scan from case 22.A showing low attenuation change involving the left temporal, frontal, and frontoparietal regions, left basal ganglia, left caudate nucleus, and left internal capsule.

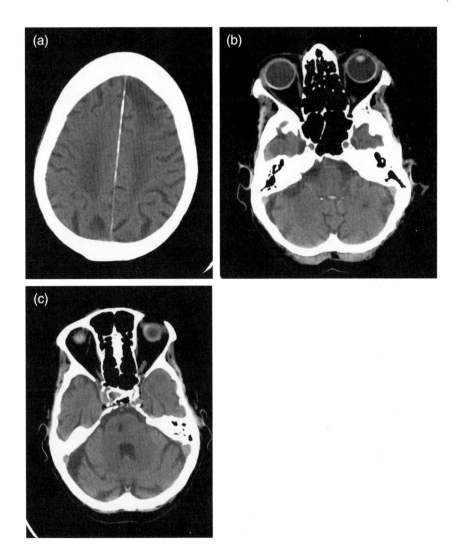

Fig. 22.2 CT brain from case 22.B showing white matter changes and a low attenuation lesion in the anterior portion of the left corona radiata compatible with an infarct (a). There is also an infarct in the left cerebellar hemisphere (b) and the right side of the pons (c).

Answers

1. What is the likely aetiology of all the cerebral ischaemic events in the two cases outlined above?

In around one-third of patients with recent ischaemic stroke or TIA, no cause is identified despite thorough diagnostic evaluation. Such patients are denoted as having 'cryptogenic stroke' and are heterogeneous in terms of risk factors, comorbid conditions, and radiographic findings. Patients who are initially diagnosed with cryptogenic stroke or TIA may subsequently be found to have intermittent AF, as in the cases illustrated here. An optimal telemetry monitoring method for the detection of occult AF could identify stroke patients at risk for recurrent cardioembolic stroke and a subgroup that may benefit from anticoagulation.

Paroxysmal AF (PAF) is believed to carry the same stroke risk as continuous AF. However, patients with PAF exhibit a wide spectrum of AF frequency and duration that may result in different risks of thromboembolism. PAF is inherently difficult to recognize and few studies have reported on telemetry monitoring methods for AF detection. A systematic review of Holter monitoring (24–72 hours) during inpatient hospitalization after ischaemic stroke has shown that the detection rate of new AF by this method is around 5%. Detection rates are higher with more prolonged monitoring. Ambulatory outpatient monitoring for 21 days detects short (minutes to hours) non-sustained AF in over 20% of patients with cryptogenic stroke, and rates are higher still in those with frequent atrial premature beats (APB) (>70 APBs).

Cardiac pacemakers have recently provided new insights into the significance of short non-sustained AF through prolonged monitoring. Non-sustained AF for >5 minutes appears to be an independent predictor of subsequent non-fatal stroke, sustained AF, and death. However, low AF burden (<5.5 hours) in a given month is reportedly associated with a low risk of thromboembolism in that month, suggesting that stroke risk is a quantitative function of PAF burden.

2. Would you have managed these patients differently prior to their most recent admissions when AF was discovered?

At present there are no clear guidelines regarding cardiac monitoring in cryptogenic stroke. Where no cause for a stroke is found after routine investigations, it remains unclear how far to continue to investigate. It would certainly seem reasonable to carry out 24-hour Holter monitoring but, as shown above, the yield is low.

3. What are the factors associated with increased risk of AF?

Factors that are associated with increased risk of AF include:

◆ older age
◆ hypertension
◆ ischaemic heart disease
◆ excess alcohol consumption

◆ cardiomyopathy

◆ hyperthyroidism.

Many of the risk factors for stroke are also risk factors for AF (e.g. older age, hypertension). AF is certainly more likely to occur in those with cardiomegaly and abnormal ECG.

4. What secondary preventive therapy would you advise?

Both patients should be anticoagulated, assuming no contraindications.

Non-rheumatic AF is by far the most common cause of cardioembolic stroke, but it cannot cause more than one-sixth of all ischaemic strokes since it is present in this proportion of ischaemic stroke patients except in the very elderly, where its prevalence is highest. The average absolute risk of stroke in non-anticoagulated non-rheumatic AF patients without prior stroke is about 4% per year, five to six times greater than in those with sinus rhythm. The risk is much higher again in patients with rheumatic AF.

The stroke risk associated with AF in an individual patient is higher in the presence of a previous embolic event, increasing age, hypertension, diabetes, left ventricular dysfunction, and an enlarged left atrium. The best validated of the stroke risk stratification schemes is the $CHADS_2$ score which awards one point each for **C**ongestive heart failure, **H**ypertension, **A**ge ≥75 years, and **D**iabetes mellitus, and 2 points for prior **S**troke or TIA. Patients with a $CHADS_2$ score of zero have a stroke risk of 0.5% per year whilst those with a score of 6 have a yearly stroke risk of 15% or more.

PAF carries the same stroke risk as persistent AF and should be treated similarly. There is no evidence that conversion to sinus rhythm followed by pharmacotherapy to try and maintain such rhythm is superior to rate control in terms of mortality and stroke risk.

Some of the association between AF and stroke must be coincidental because AF can be caused by coronary and hypertensive heart disease, both of which may be associated with atheromatous disease or primary ICH. Although anticoagulation markedly reduces the risk of first or recurrent stroke, this is not necessarily evidence for causality because this treatment may be working in other ways, such as by inhibiting artery-to-artery embolism, although trials of warfarin in secondary prevention of stroke in sinus rhythm have shown no benefit over aspirin (see below).

Therefore patients in AF who have a TIA or stroke without other clear aetiology should be anticoagulated if there are no contraindications. Recent trials (Birmingham Atrial Fibrillation Treatment of the Aged Study (BAFTA), Warfarin versus Aspirin for Stroke Prevention in Octogenarians with AF (WASPO)) have shown that warfarin is as safe as aspirin in elderly patients with AF. Patients with presumed cardioembolic TIA or stroke secondary to other causes should certainly receive antithrombotic therapy. They may also benefit from anticoagulation in certain circumstances, such as intracardiac mural thrombosis after myocardial infarction, although there have been no randomized trials in situations other than non-valvular AF.

Anticoagulation is not effective in secondary prevention of stroke for patients in sinus rhythm. Warfarin treatment to a target international normalized ratio (INR) of 3–4.5 was associated with significant harm because of a large increase in major bleeding complications, especially ICH, in patients with previous TIA or ischaemic stroke in the SPIRIT trial. The subsequent WARSS Trial of aspirin versus warfarin for patients in sinus rhythm and without a cardioembolic source or >50% carotid stenosis showed no additional benefit for warfarin at a target INR of 1.4–2.8.

Patients who are felt to be at high risk of bleeding complications or falls, or with suspected CAA and previous ICH (see Case 6), should receive aspirin. Warfarin may also be problematic in patients unable to manage the regular blood tests and dose adjustments that warfarin therapy requires. Newer drugs such as dabigatran (anticoagulants that do not require regular blood test monitoring) may become the future mainstay of therapy for secondary prevention of stroke for those in AF.

Further reading

Blackshear JL, Safford RE (2003). AFFIRM and RACE trials: implications for the management of atrial fibrillation. *Cardiol Electrophys Rev*; **7**: 366–9.

European Atrial Fibrillation Trial Study Group (1993). Secondary prevention in non-rheumatic atrial fibrillation after transient ischaemic attack or minor stroke. *Lancet* **342**: 1255–62.

European Atrial Fibrillation Trial Study Group (1995). Optimal oral anticoagulant therapy in patients with nonrheumatic atrial fibrillation and recent cerebral ischemia. *N Engl J Med*; **333**: 5–10.

Gaillard N, Deltour S, Vilotijevic B, *et al.* (2010). Detection of paroxysmal atrial fibrillation with transtelephonic EKG in TIA or stroke patients. *Neurology*; **74**: 1666–70.

Glotzer TV, Hellkamp AS, Zimmerman J, *et al.* (2003). Atrial high rate episodes detected by pacemaker diagnostics predict death and stroke: report of the atrial diagnostics ancillary study of the Mode Selection Trial (MOST). *Circulation*; **107**: 1614–19.

Glotzer TV, Daoud EG, Wyse G, *et al.* (2009). The relationship between daily atrial tachyarrhythmia burden from implantable device diagnostics and stroke risk: the TRENDS Study. *Circ Arrhythmia Electrophysiol*; **2**: 474–80.

Jabaudon D, Sztajzel J, Sievert K, Landis T, Sztajzel R (2004). Usefulness of ambulatory 7-day ECG monitoring for detection of atrial fibrillation and flutter after acute stroke and transient ischemic attack. *Stroke*; **35**: 1647–51.

Liao J, Khalid Z, Scallan C, Morillo C, O'Donnell M (2007). Noninvasive cardiac monitoring for detecting paroxysmal atrial fibrillation or flutter after acute ischemic stroke: a systematic review. *Stroke*; **38**: 2935–40.

Mant J, Hobbs FD, Fletcher K, *et al.* (2007). Warfarin versus aspirin for stroke prevention in an elderly community population with atrial fibrillation (the Birmingham Atrial Fibrillation Treatment of the Aged Study, BAFTA): a randomised controlled trial. *Lancet*; **370**: 493–503.

Rash A, Downes T, Portner R, Yeo WW, Morgan N, Channer KS (2007). A randomised controlled trial of warfarin versus aspirin for stroke prevention in octogenarians with atrial fibrillation (WASPO). *Age Ageing*; **36**: 151–6.

Tayal AH, Tian M, Kelly KM, *et al.* (2008). Atrial fibrillation detected by mobile cardiac outpatient telemetry in cryptogenic stroke or TIA. *Neurology*; **71**: 1696–1701.

Wallman D, Tuller D, Wustmann K, *et al.* (2007). Frequent atrial premature beats predict paroxysmal atrial fibrillation in stroke patients: an opportunity for a new diagnostic strategy. *Stroke*; **38**: 2292–4.

Case 23

A 54-year-old woman presented with a history of three episodes of left-sided numbness and weakness over the preceding 2 months. She described 'tingling and throbbing' which started in the sole of her left foot and gradually spread up the left leg and trunk, into the left arm, and down into the hand. This occurred over several minutes. By the time the tingling started in her left hand, it had subsided in her foot. For some hours after an episode she noticed her left arm and leg feeling heavy and possibly weak. She had not had any blackouts.

Questions

1. What is the most likely diagnosis? Give a differential diagnosis.
2. Describe the radiological features of the CT and MRI scans (Figs 23.1 and 23.2). What is the diagnosis?
3. Describe common presenting features of the type of lesion shown on the scan.
4. What are the main subtypes of of the condition given as your answer for Question 1, and its causes?
5. What advice would you give such patients regarding driving?

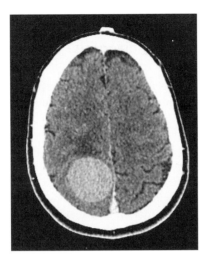

Fig. 23.1 CT brain.

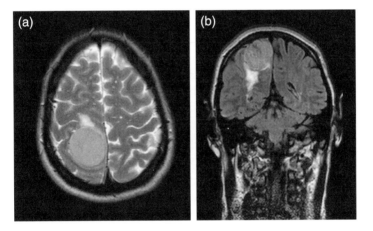

Fig. 23.2 MRI brain: axial T2-weighted image (a) and coronal FLAIR image (b).

Answers

1. What is the most likely diagnosis? Give a differential diagnosis

The most likely diagnosis is focal epileptic seizures. The differential diagnosis of recurrent stereotyped hemisensory symptoms includes recurrent cerebrovascular events, migraine with aura (see Case 7), demyelination (see Case 13), space-occupying lesions (see Case 1), and functional disorders (see Case 20).

Simple partial seizures can present with motor, sensory, visual, or autonomic symptoms, depending on which part of the brain the abnormal electrical discharges arise from. Sensory seizures often present with a 'march' of symptoms, i.e. the sensory disturbance begins in one part of the body and gradually spreads to other parts, for example from the foot up the leg as in the patient we have described. Equally, motor seizures may begin with repeated jerking movements of the hand, which then gradually spread to involve the entire arm and ipsilateral side of the face. The spread of symptoms reflects the spread of electrical activity in the cortex. Focal motor seizures may be followed by weakness of the affected limb. This is called Todd's palsy (see Case 42). It reflects a postictal refractory period during which the cortical motor neurons are unable to fire sufficiently to initiate movement. This period usually lasts for some minutes, but sometimes requires some days to resolve, and it is sometimes mistakenly diagnosed as being due to a vascular event. Therefore in patients presenting with limb weakness, it is important to ask whether any involuntary movements or limb jerking preceded the onset of the weakness and to elicit whether there have ever been any previous focal seizures to help differentiate an ischaemic event from Todd's palsy.

2. Describe the radiological features of the CT and MRI scans (Figs 23.1 and 23.2). What is the diagnosis?

Figure 23.1 shows a well-demarcated round mass in the right parieto-occipital region. There is bright regular enhancement after giving contrast. The most likely diagnosis is a meningioma. This diagnosis is further supported by the findings on the MRI scan (Fig. 23.2) which shows a well-demarcated round lesion which appears to arise from the meninges (Fig. 23.2(a)), and which has some peri-lesional oedema (Fig. 23.2(b)) although very little space-occupying effect.

MRI has largely superseded CT as the imaging modality of choice for brain tumours. Not only does it allow a more detailed assessment of the tumour and its relationship to the surrounding parenchyma, but it is also superior for evaluation of the meninges, subarachnoid space, and posterior fossa, and for defining the vascular supply to a tumour. In addition, other sequences, such as MR spectroscopy, also allow the metabolic activity of tumours to be assessed and the tumour to be graded to at least some extent even before a biopsy is taken. The main advantages of CT are its more widespread availability, especially in an emergency setting. Furthermore, it is also helpful in detecting any bony lesions, in particular metastases affecting the skull base. Finally, CT provides vital information in those patients in whom MRI is contraindicated (e.g. those with cardiac pacemakers).

Table 23.1 Locations for meningiomas and associated symptoms

Location	Symptoms
Parasagittal	Monoparesis of contralateral leg
Subfrontal	Change in behaviour, disinhibition, urinary incontinence
Olfactory groove	Anosmia with possible ipsilateral optic atrophy and contralateral papilloedema (Foster–Kennedy syndrome)
Cavernous sinus	Multiple CN deficits (CN II–VI)
Occipital lobe	Contralateral homonymous hemianopia
Cerebellopontine angle	Decreased hearing with possible facial weakness and numbness
Spinal cord	Localized spinal pain, Brown–Sequard syndrome

3. Describe common presenting features of the type of lesion shown on the scan.

The scan appearances are highly suggestive of a meningioma. Meningiomas arise from the meninges and therefore are not 'brain' tumours, but they may still cause seizures by irritating the underlying cortex. They may also cause a variety of other symptoms by compressing the brain or cranial nerves, producing hyperostosis, and invading surrounding soft tissues or inducing vascular injuries to the brain. There are some locations in which meningiomas occur relatively frequently, and they may then cause fairly specific symptoms. Common locations for meningiomas and frequently associated symptoms are listed in Table 23.1.

4. What are the main subtypes of the condition given as your answer to Question 1, and its causes?

Seizures are classified according to whether the source of the seizure within the brain is localized (**partial** or **focal** onset seizures) or not related to localization (**generalized** seizures). Partial seizures are further categorized, depending on the extent to which consciousness is affected, into **simple partial** seizures, in which full consciousness is preserved, and **complex partial** seizures, with impaired consciousness. The initially localized electrical disturbance that causes a focal seizure may spread within the brain—a process known as **secondary generalization**.

The symptoms caused by focal seizures depend on the location of the underlying lesion. For example, tumours in the motor cortex may cause focal tonic–clonic movements involving a single limb. Seizures originating within the occipital lobe may cause visual disturbances. A typical presentation of occipital lobe seizures is the perception of coloured circles in the affected visual hemifield. Temporal lobe seizures can cause behavioural disturbances, with or without auras (e.g. abnormal smell, taste, or *déjà-vu* phenomena).

Focal seizures can be caused by any localized structural lesion within the cerebral cortex, but also by some systemic abnormalities. Such causes include:

◆ vascular lesions
◆ meningitis/focal encephalitis

- trauma
- developmental abnormalities
- intracerebral neoplasms
- hypoxic brain injury
- metabolic and electrolyte shifts
- hippocampal sclerosis.

Generalized seizures are generally divided into primary and secondary generalized seizures. Secondary generalized seizures are due to an underlying focal lesion. There is often a history of focal onset, and they are the most common type of generalized seizure occurring in adulthood. Primary generalized seizures often occur from childhood onwards. They are often associated with genetic defects and underlying channelopathies. Examples of primary generalized seizures include childhood absences or juvenile myoclonic epilepsy.

5. What advice would you give such patients regarding driving?

Driving regulations for patients with seizures and with epilepsy differ between countries. In the UK, patients must stop driving with immediate effect with all types of seizures, even without a diagnosis of epilepsy. The doctor must inform the patient of the driving regulations for seizures, but it is the patient's responsibility to inform the Driver and Vehicle Licensing Agency (DVLA) and to return their driving license. If a diagnosis of epilepsy is made, a patient will have to remain seizure-free for 1 year before they can drive again. For large goods vehicles, patients have to be seizure-free for 10 years.

Patients who suffered a first and single seizure only may start driving after 6 months following assessment by a specialist if no relevant abnormality is found on investigation (e.g. EEG, MRI head), they have no further seizures, and they meet all the standard requirements to drive. The driving restriction for large goods vehicle drivers is 5 years.

Patients with benign brain tumours in the brainstem and cerebellum can drive again as soon as their treatment is completed. If the benign brain tumour is elsewhere in the brain, patients cannot drive for a year. The exception is a benign meningioma, for which patients may be allowed to drive again after 6 months if seizure-free. Latest guidance is available at www.dft.gov.uk/dvla.

Further reading

Driver and Vehicle Licensing Authority. *At a Glance Guide to the Current Medical Standards of Fitness to Drive*: www.dft.gov.uk/dvla/medical/ataglance.aspx.

Werhahn KJ (2010). Weakness and focal sensory deficits in the postictal state. *Epilepsy Behav*; **19**: 138–9.

Case 24

A 16-year-old boy skidded on a puddle while riding his motorbike. He fell and hit his head, but had been wearing a helmet, did not lose consciousness, and had no post-traumatic amnesia. The next morning, after having been observed in hospital overnight, he noticed that his left arm felt slightly numb and heavy. This was attributed to some bruising, and as he was otherwise well, he was discharged home. Some hours later, while watching TV, he suddenly complained of feeling unwell and a few moments later collapsed. He did not lose consciousness, but appeared vague. His parents noted slurred speech and a left-sided facial and arm weakness. They took their son back to the accident and emergency department where, on examination, pupillary asymmetry was found in addition to the left-sided weakness and sensory loss. There was no hemianopia and no neglect. The patient was admitted and a CT brain scan was organized (Fig. 24.1).

The next day, the patient appeared more drowsy. Although he remained orientated and obeyed commands, he only opened his eyes to speech.

Questions

1. What is the likely diagnosis?
2. What is the pupillary asymmetry due to? Which pupil was smaller?
3. What does the CT brain scan (Fig. 24.1) show? What is the white dot pointed out by the arrow?
4. Which further imaging would you arrange? Discuss the different available modalities.
5. Which medication, if any, would you give this patient?
6. What potential complication in this young stroke patient would you be worried about?
7. Which intervention should be considered in patients who develop this complication?

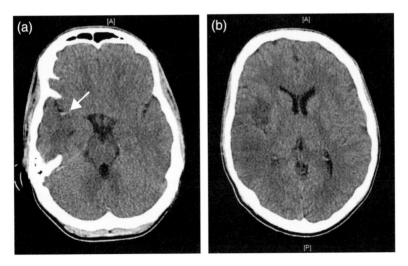

Fig. 24.1 CT brain scan on transfer, 1 day after symptom onset and 2 days after the accident.

Answers

1. What is the likely diagnosis?

The most likely diagnosis is an ischaemic stroke due to a traumatic carotid artery dissection. Given the history of head injury, one should not forget the possibility of a traumatic extradural or subdural haematoma. However, after a minor head injury without loss of consciousness or amnesia, it is very unlikely that such a complication would develop. Furthermore, the symptom onset appears too sudden for an extradural or subdural haematoma and would be more in keeping with an embolic event.

2. What is the pupillary asymmetry due to? Which pupil was smaller?

The pupillary asymmetry is due to Horner's syndrome. This is caused by interruption of the sympathetic fibres in the wall of the dissected carotid artery. As the patient has a left hemiparesis, he probably has a right-sided carotid dissection and right-sided Horner's syndrome, i.e. his right pupil will be smaller. Although the classical triad for Horner's syndrome is miosis, ptosis, and enophthalmos, this is often incomplete with only the pupillary abnormality being noticeable.

3. What does the CT brain scan (Fig. 24.1) show? What is the white dot pointed out by the arrow?

The CT brain scan shows an established infarct in the right lentiform nucleus (b), with slightly less obvious ischaemic changes also visible in the middle and posterior MCA territory. The white dot in (a) represents fresh thrombus in the middle cerebral artery as it runs through the Sylvian fissure, an example of the 'hyperdense MCA sign', which can often be found in patients with acute ischaemic stroke.

4. Which further imaging would you arrange? Discuss the different available modalities.

The presentation strongly suggests a traumatic carotid artery dissection. Vascular imaging is indicated to confirm this diagnosis, exclude other diagnoses, determine the extent of the dissection, and assess whether it has led to vessel occlusion or stenosis, which may determine the risk of further embolic events. Several imaging modalities are available. Doppler ultrasound is easily available, but only offers a limited view of the carotid artery and is operator dependent. Classically, intra-arterial digital subtraction angiography (DSA) has been regarded as the gold standard for diagnosing cervical artery dissection. Features may include a tapering occlusion, an intimal flap, an irregular stenosis, or a double lumen. However, as DSA carries a risk of complications, it is no longer done routinely. MRI and MRA are non-invasive and are now accepted as an alternative to DSA. In addition to appearances on the MRA, the presence of an intramural haematoma supports the diagnosis of an arterial dissection. As the haematoma may be difficult to differentiate from surrounding perivascular fat, a T1-weighted fat-suppression technique should be used.

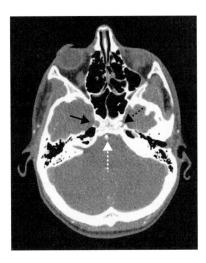

Fig. 24.2 CTA showing the right carotid occlusion (solid black arrow). The vessel does not fill with contrast, whereas contrast is clearly visible in the left carotid artery (black dashed arrow) and the basilar artery (white dashed arrow).

Finally CTA is a further imaging technique, possibly more sensitive than MRI/MRA, but it has the disadvantages of having to use contrast and a high radiation dose. In our patient, we used CTA for further vascular imaging. This showed an occlusive dissection of the right ICA, starting 2.7 cm from the origin and extending to the cavernous portion of the carotid siphon (Fig. 24.2).

5. Which medication, if any, would you give this patient?

Treatment in this patient should be directed at trying to reduce the damage caused by the current infarction and at preventing further events. At the time of review, the patient was already well outside the time window for thrombolysis. There has been some debate as to whether thrombolysis in acute cervical artery dissection may carry a higher risk than in other types of ischaemic stroke, given the presence of a haematoma in the vessel wall. Current available data suggest that thrombolysis in these patients carries the same risk as in other types of stroke, but there are no data on the efficacy of thrombolysis in this patient group. To prevent further embolic events from a cervical artery dissection, either antiplatelet agents or anticoagulants have been used. A recent systematic review found no difference in stroke risk or complication rate between these treatments. However, no reliable prospective randomized data are available. A randomized controlled trial (CADISS: www.dissection.co.uk) addressing this question is now under way. A further option to prevent recurrent events and to treat stenotic lesions and dissecting aneurysms may be stenting. Although this has a high technical success rate, its efficacy in preventing further events is currently unclear. The risk of further embolic events appeared relatively low in our patient, as the carotid artery was occluded. There was also a fairly large area of established infarction already. Therefore the risk of causing an intracranial haemorrhage when using anticoagulation appeared high, and we decided to use aspirin for secondary prevention.

6. What potential complication in this young stroke patient would you be worried about?

Malignant MCA infarction—a large cerebral infarct, as in this patient, will cause swelling. In a young patient with no cerebral atrophy, this may lead to increased intracranial pressure and cause midline shift and tentorial herniation, which are potentially life-threatening complications.

7. Which intervention should be considered in patients who develop this complication?

Decompressive hemicraniectomy: during this procedure, a large part of the skull bone is removed. This allows the brain to swell without causing midline shift or brainstem compression. Once the swelling has gone down, the bone may be replaced or the bony defect can be covered with a titanium plate. The benefit of this procedure has been much debated, as the fear was that patients with a severe stroke, who would otherwise die, might survive but be severely disabled. However, an individual patient data meta-analysis of three randomized trials showed beneficial results if decompressive craniectomy was performed within 48 hours of cerebral infarction, with a number needed to treat (NNT) of 2 for survival irrespective of outcome, NNT of 2 for survival with a modified Rankin Scale (mRS) score ≤4, and NNT of 4 for survival with an mRS score ≤3. As our patient had not infarcted his whole MCA territory, decompression was originally withheld. However, he then became increasingly drowsy, and follow-up scanning on day 3 after the infarct showed significant midline shift (Fig. 24.3). Decompressive craniectomy was performed, but did not lead to an improvement in level of consciousness or shift (Fig. 24.4). Therefore contralateral craniectomy was performed the next day (Fig. 24.5). The patient then began to improve. On transfer back to his local hospital, he was alert and orientated and only had a mild left hemiparesis.

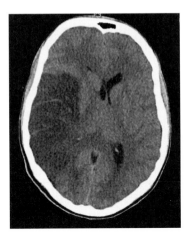

Fig. 24.3 Midline shift after right-sided MCA infarction.

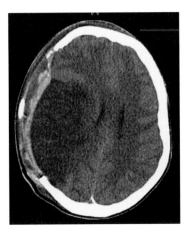

Fig. 24.4 Persisting midline shift and swelling after right-sided decompressive hemicraniectomy.

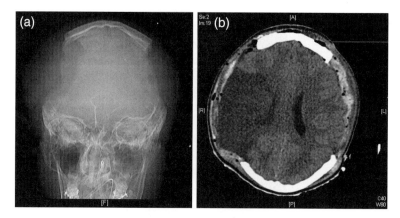

Fig. 24.5 (a) Scout image showing the bony defects after bilateral decompressive hemicraniectomy. (b) Persisting swelling, but no more midline shift after bilateral decompressive hemicraniectomy.

Further reading

Goyal MS, Derdeyn CP (2009). The diagnosis and management of supraaortic arterial dissections. *Curr Opin Neurol*; **22**: 80–9.

Menon R, Kerry S, Norris JW, Markus HS (2008). Treatment of cervical artery dissection: a systematic review and meta-analysis. *J Neurol Neurosurg Psych*; **79**: 1122–7.

Vahedi K, Hofmeijer J, Juettler E, *et al.* (2007). Early decompressive surgery in malignant infarction of the middle cerebral artery: a pooled analysis of three randomised controlled trials. *Lancet Neurol*; **6**: 215–22.

Case 25

A 34-year-old Nigerian woman presented with sudden-onset confusion and collapse. Two months previously, she had been admitted with headache, fever, and raised inflammatory markers. At that time, blood and urine cultures and CT head, chest, abdomen, and pelvis had been unremarkable, and a lumbar puncture had shown slightly elevated protein but no cells. There was a past history of SLE diagnosed 5 years previously following a cheek ulcer, and depression with suicidal ideation a year before this admission. Medications included prednisolone, azathioprine, and mirtazapine.

On arrival in the emergency department, she was very confused but there was no focal neurological deficit. The following morning, she had a focal seizure affecting the right arm and face that terminated spontaneously. She was subsequently noted to have a right-sided weakness with receptive and expressive dysphasia.

DWI and MRA brain are shown in Figs 25.1 and 25.2, respectively.

Questions

1. What do the DWI (Fig. 25.1) and the intracranial MRA (Fig. 25.2) show?
2. What are the factors predisposing to seizures in this case?
3. What is the likely cause of her stroke? Is her past medical history relevant?

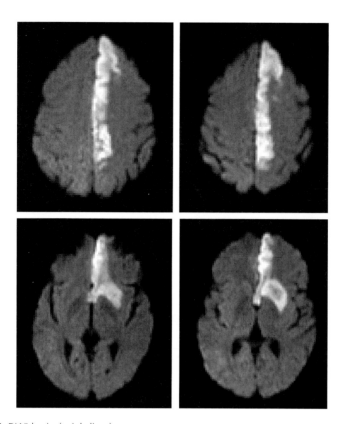

Fig. 25.1 DWI brain (axial slices).

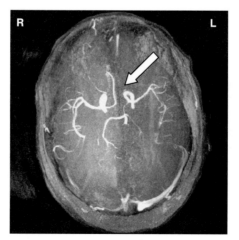

Fig. 25.2 Intracranial MRA.

Answers

1. What do the DWI (Fig. 25.1) and the intracranial MRA (Fig. 25.2) show?

The DWI shows high signal in the left frontal lobe, mainly involving the cortex of the superior frontal gyrus and the interhemispheric surface, but also the straight gyrus, as well as the caudate nucleus. (Fig. 25.1) There is also high signal on the T2-weighted images (Fig. 25.3). Appearances are in keeping with acute infarction affecting the left anterior cerebral artery (ACA) territory, including the territory of the recurrent artery of Heubner. This infarct pattern would be unusual for an embolic event, as the embolus would have to be big enough to occlude both the origin of Heubner's artery, which normally branches off the ACA proximal to the anterior communicating artery, and the origin of the anterior communicating artery, which would otherwise provide collateral flow to the remainder of the ACA territory. An inflammatory aetiology may be more likely. The MRA (Fig. 25.2) shows an occluded left ACA (arrow) and irregular narrowing (beading) of left MCA and PCA branches.

2. What are the factors predisposing to seizures in this case?

The factors predisposing to seizures in this case are:

♦ the presence of a large area of cortical infarction

♦ antidepressant use

♦ underlying cerebral metabolic abnormality secondary to SLE.

The prevalence of seizures after stroke is highest in the immediate post-stroke period at around 5% and reaches around 10% at 5 years. Seizures are more likely after haemorrhage and after large cortical infarcts. Cerebrovascular disease is the most common cause of new-onset seizures in the elderly, and apparently idiopathic seizures occurring *de novo* in elderly subjects are associated with an increased risk of subsequent stroke.

This patient had been prescribed antidepressants for severe psychotic depression. Antidepressants cause a reduction in seizure threshold and therefore will

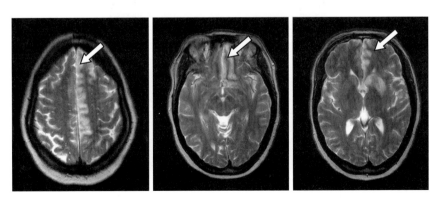

Fig. 25.3 T2-weighted images.

increase the likelihood of seizures after cerebral injury. The presence of confusion in the absence of focal neurology at the time of presentation suggests an element of encephalopathy which is also associated with increased seizure risk.

3. What is the likely cause of her stroke? Is her past medical history relevant?

The most likely cause of the stroke is large vessel vasculitis associated with SLE.

The most likely diagnosis is of a large vessel vasculitis/vasculopathy with associated infarction. A beaded appearance of the cerebral vessels may occur in vasculitis (see also Case 11) reversible cerebral vasoconstriction syndrome (RCVS) (see Case 34) and IVBCL (see Case 50).

Although vasculitis is often assumed to be the cause of stroke in patients with SLE, in fact there is often little evidence in support of this aetiology. Angiographic findings may be suggestive of vasculitis, but autopsy series have failed to provide much evidence. Vasculopathy with perivascular inflammatory infiltrates and haemorrhage seems more common. Cardiogenic stroke may occur secondary to Libman–Sacks endocarditis. Hypercoagulable states may also predispose to stroke. The lupus anticoagulant and anticardiolipin antibodies are associated with venous thromboembolism, spontaneous abortion, and stroke. These antibodies were initially described in association with SLE, but may also occur in its absence. Atherosclerosis may be more frequent in those with SLE because of the use of steroids, resulting in an altered lipid profile and immunological abnormalities.

SLE may also cause a diffuse encephalopathy with a normal MRI scan. In the current patient, it is likely that the episode of pyrexia and headache that occurred a few weeks prior to the current presentation was caused by a flare in the activity of her SLE. At that time her CRP was elevated and complement levels were low with high levels of dsDNA. Further, the episode of psychotic depression that occurred a year before in the absence of any prior history of depression was also probably a manifestation of SLE, as psychosis is another common feature of cerebral lupus.

The episode of headache followed by confusion and focal neurological deficit with beading on the MRA could be consistent with RCVS (see Case 34). However, this diagnosis is less likely in view of the fact that the patient recovered and was back at work before becoming unwell with confusion, whereas RCVS usually presents as a monophasic illness. Headache and neurological deficit in someone with a history of SLE may also be caused by venous sinus thrombosis (see Case 17).

The patient had a good response to immunosuppressive therapy in terms of her SLE activity and made a reasonable neurological recovery. However, although she recovered independent mobility, she was left with significant cognitive impairment including attentional and executive deficits requiring prompting for all but the simplest tasks. Cognitive impairment after stroke is associated with a number of stroke-related factors including the size of the infarct (see Case 8). The fact that this patient's brain was probably globally abnormal secondary to SLE with metabolic and widespread vascular changes meant that there was increased vulnerability to the effects of stroke and less capacity for recovery. Attentional and executive deficits are the most common cognitive abnormalities detected early after stroke and predict poor functional and cognitive outcome.

Further reading

Chaves CJ (2004). Stroke in patients with systemic lupus erythematosus and antiphospholipid antibody syndrome. *Curr Treat Options Cardiovasc Med*; **6**: 223–9.

Devinsky O, Petito CK, Alonso DR (1988). Clinical and neuropathological findings in systemic lupus erythematosus: the role of vasculitis, heart emboli and thrombotic thrombocytopenic purpura. *Ann Neurol*; **23**: 380–4.

Futrell N, Millikan C (1989). Frequency, etiology, and prevention of stroke in patients with systemic lupus erythematosus. *Stroke*; **20**: 583–91.

Futrell N, Schulz LR, Millikan C (1992). Central nervous system disease in patients with systemic lupus erythematosus. *Neurology*; **42**: 1649–57.

Ishimori ML, Pressman BD, Wallace DJ, Weisman MH (2007). Posterior reversible encephalopathy syndrome: another manifestation of CNS SLE? *Lupus*; **16**: 436–43.

Mikdashi J, Krumholz A, Handwerger B (2005). Factors at diagnosis predict subsequent occurrence of seizures in systemic lupus erythematosus. *Neurology*; **64**: 2102–7.

Mitsias P, Levine SR (1994). Large cerebral vessel occlusive disease in systemic lupus erythematosus. *Neurology*; **44**: 385–93.

Case 26

Case 26.A

A 73-year-old woman presented to the accident and emergency department. She had recently been diagnosed with diabetes, and had followed her family practitioner's encouragement to lose some weight. She also had a history of mild hypertension, but was otherwise healthy. She had woken up in the morning with difficulty walking, and noticed that she found it difficult to lift her right foot. She reported no pain and no sensory disturbance. Her right arm, vision, and speech were normal. Clinical examination revealed a right foot drop and weak ankle inversion and eversion. There was no sensory deficit. Reflexes were symmetrical, with bilaterally absent ankle jerks. Plantar responses were flexor. Blood pressure was 160/90mmHg.

Case 26.B

A 55-year-old man was found lying in the street. He was confused, but able to state that he had been on his way home from visiting a friend some hours earlier. Examination in the emergency department revealed a bruise on the forehead and a bitten tongue. The patient was poorly cooperative, but he was obviously using his right arm less than his left. A CT brain scan was difficult to interpret because of movement artefact, but showed no obvious abnormality apart from atrophy. The patient was observed overnight. The next morning he was alert and orientated, but had no recollections from the night before. He admitted to regular heavy alcohol consumption, but stated that he had drastically reduced this some days previously. He was also a smoker, and had had a previous myocardial infarction. He was now able to cooperate with the examination. This revealed weakness of right wrist and finger extension. There was also some sensory loss in the right forearm. Reflexes were symmetrical. Face, leg, speech, and vision were normal.

Questions

1. What is the differential diagnosis in patient A? And in patient B?
2. How would you investigate these patients further?
3. How would you treat these patients?

Answers

1. What is the differential diagnosis in patient A? And in patient B?

The main differential diagnosis in patient A is between a right common peroneal nerve palsy and a stroke in the left anterior cerebral artery territory. While an L5 root lesion is also possible, there is nothing in the history suggesting any back problems, and in an acute root lesion, especially in root compression, one would expect at least some pain. As the onset of the patient's symptoms was overnight, it is impossible to tell if symptom onset was sudden, as would be expected in a stroke. Certainly, the patient's age and her history of diabetes and hypertension would put her at risk of having an ischaemic event. However, the patient's recent weight loss would also put her at risk of nerve compression at the fibular head, and her diabetes may make her more susceptible to developing a common peroneal nerve palsy.

History and examination findings in patient B strongly suggest that he has had a generalized seizure. Therefore one might expect an intracranial process as the cause of his right arm weakness. This could be due to Todd's palsy (see also Case 42) or a vascular event, which would not necessarily be visible on a poor-quality CT scan. A further differential is that the patient had a generalized seizure, possibly brought on by alcohol withdrawal. During the subsequent period of unconsciousness and postictal sleep, he may have compressed his radial nerve, leading to his right wrist drop.

2. How would you investigate these patients further?

In both patients, the main differential diagnosis is between an acute peripheral nerve lesion and a cerebrovascular event. Both patients have risk factors for both conditions, and there is insufficient history available about the symptom onset to help with the diagnosis. Clinical examination is not particularly helpful in either patient. The two main investigations which should help with making the diagnosis are nerve conduction studies and brain imaging, preferably MRI brain with diffusion-weighted imaging to show recent ischaemia, and GRE to show haemorrhage. In a compressive nerve lesion, nerve conduction studies should show conduction block at the site of the compression. Denervation on electromyography will only show up after a delay of 1–2 weeks, and therefore is not necessarily helpful in the acute stage. Further investigations would then depend on the diagnosis. Patient A was found to have a small left anterior cerebral artery infarct. Her further investigations should be directed at determining stroke aetiology and treatable risk factors. She should have imaging of the cervical and possibly intracranial arteries with either Doppler ultrasound, MRA or CTA. She should also have an ECG to look for an arrhythmia, potentially echocardiography to look for a cardioembolic source, and blood tests, including full blood count, inflammatory markers, cholesterol, and, as she is known to be diabetic, HbA1c.

Patient B turned out to have a right radial nerve palsy with a conduction block in the right upper arm, most likely due to having compressed his radial nerve for a prolonged time after his seizure. In the first instance, the radial nerve palsy would not require further investigation, although this would have to be reconsidered if the patient developed further neuropathies. However, even with the arm weakness explained, the patient should still have good-quality brain imaging, preferably MRI, if this was his first seizure. While alcohol withdrawal may be the most likely aetiology, a first seizure at the age of 55 years warrants brain imaging to look for an underlying structural lesion. The patient's MRI confirmed atrophy and mild small vessel disease, but showed no other abnormality. An EEG is not essential, as there is not much doubt about the diagnosis of a seizure, imaging showed no suspicious lesions, and the aetiology appears to be explained.

Both these cases demonstrate that occasionally it can be difficult or impossible to differentiate between a peripheral nerve lesion and a cerebrovascular event. Reasons include an insufficient history and the fact that physical signs may be misleading or unhelpful. In particular in the acute stage, it may be difficult to differentiate between central and peripheral lesions. If in doubt, all diagnostic possibilities should be explored.

3. How would you treat these patients?

Further investigations of patient A revealed no significant vascular stenosis and no cardioembolic source. If there are no contraindications, she should be treated with antiplatelet drugs, either a combination of aspirin and slow-release dipyridamole or clopidogrel as a single antiplatelet agent. She should also be started on a statin, and her blood pressure management and diabetic control should be optimized.

Patient B may require physiotherapy and a splint for his wrist. Acutely, he may require management of alcohol withdrawal, and should also be given high-dose thiamine to prevent Wernicke's encephalopathy. In the longer term, he should receive counselling and help for his alcohol abuse. As this was his first seizure, and as it was provoked, he would not usually require anti-epileptic drugs, in particular as compliance might be an issue. The patient stated that he was driving a car occasionally. As he had had a single alcohol-related seizure, his licence will be revoked for a minimum of 6 months. The DVLA also regulates alcohol misuse, which leads to licence revocation until a minimum 6-month period of controlled drinking or abstinence has been achieved. Alcohol dependency leads to licence revocation until at least a year free from alcohol problems has been achieved. The patient should be alerted to these regulations.

Further reading

DVLA *At a glance guide to the current medical standards to drive*, pp.37–8. Available online at http://www.dft.gov.uk/dvla/medical/ataglance.aspx.

Hand PJ, Kwan J, Lindley RI, *et al.* (2006). Distinguishing between stroke and mimic at the bedside: the brain attack study. *Stroke*; **37**: 769–75.

Case 27

Case 27.A

A 74-year-old man developed three episodes of sudden-onset dysarthria over a period of 4 months, each lasting 15 minutes and resolving spontaneously. He remained well between attacks. On review in the TIA clinic, examination was unremarkable. Carotid ultrasound showed minimal stenoses and brain MRI showed minor small vessel disease only.

Case 27.B

A 64-year-old man developed sudden-onset slurred speech and difficulty in swallowing. He had a past medical history of a mild ischaemic stroke 2 years previously that had caused left upper limb weakness and slurred speech, from which he had made a full recovery. He was hypertensive and hypercholesterolaemic with a strong family history of vascular disease. After several weeks, his symptoms had improved but had not fully resolved. He then had a further episode of sudden-onset swallowing difficulty and slurred speech. CT brain showed several small ischaemic lesions in the deep white matter. There was moderate carotid stenosis on carotid ultrasound.

Questions

1. Other than cerebrovascular disease, which diagnoses would you consider that could apply to the cases above?
2. What particular aspects of the clinical examination might help narrow the differential diagnosis?

Answers

1. Other than cerebrovascular disease, which diagnoses would you consider that could apply to the cases above?

Both patients developed sudden-onset speech difficulty. In both cases the episodes were recurrent, with the first patient remaining well in between episodes. The differential diagnosis in older patients excluding cerebrovascular disease is:

◆ myasthenia gravis

◆ motor neuron disease (MND) (amyotrophic lateral sclerosis (ALS))

◆ brainstem space-occupying lesion

◆ multiple sclerosis (usually in younger patients) (see Case 13).

Myasthenia gravis may present with episodic symptoms affecting one anatomical region and without a history of fatiguability. Elderly patients in particular may present with non-specific symptoms on a background of significant comorbidity, making the diagnosis difficult. Symptoms may be triggered by intercurrent illness or drugs. There is evidence that myasthenia is underdiagnosed in elderly patients. The diagnosis is supported by a positive acetylcholine receptor antibody test, EMG, and thymoma on CT thorax. There is an association with other autoimmune diseases such as hypothyroidism and Addison's disease.

Patients with MND may also present with bulbar symptoms in the absence of symptoms and signs in other areas and without tongue fasciculation, and symptoms may be episodic initially.

Multiple sclerosis causes episodic neurological symptoms which may come on suddenly, although presentation is usually subacute. Onset is usually in the third or fourth decade and is more common in women, but presentation as late as the seventh decade has been reported. There are often signs of asymptomatic disease in other areas of the nervous system (e.g. optic neuritis) and/or previous episodes of, for example, optic neuritis or transverse myelitis.

Brain imaging in elderly patients is often abnormal with ischaemic areas in the deep white matter or leukoaraiosis (confluent periventricular white matter abnormality) (see Cases 6 and 49). This may be taken to be supportive of a vascular aetiology in elderly patients presenting with TIA/minor stroke-like episodes without consideration of alternative diagnoses. Multiple sclerosis lesions may be indistinguishable from ischaemic lesions, especially in older patients. In multiple sclerosis, lesions are periventricular and typically ovoid or flame-shaped (see Case 13).

Space-occupying lesions may present with TIA/stroke-like episodes caused by haemorrhage, compressive effects of the tumour, vascular steal, or focal seizures (see Case 1). Focal seizures would be unusual in a brainstem lesion although movement disorders such as hemifacial spasm and tongue dystonia may occur (see Fig. 27.1).

Some other neurological causes of dysarthria are listed on page 159, but they do not cause episodic symptoms, being generally progressive and associated with other abnormalities.

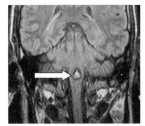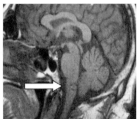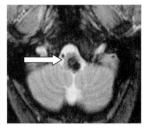

Fig. 27.1 MRI brain. This shows a cavernoma in the brainstem (arrows), which caused tongue dystonia.

- ◆ Movement disorders:
  - Parkinson's disease and Parkinson's plus syndromes
  - Wilson's disease
  - Huntingdon's disease
- ◆ Polio and post-polio syndromes
- ◆ Peripheral neuropathy:
  - Guillain–Barré syndrome
  - diphtheria
  - porphyria
- ◆ Muscle disease:
  - polymyositis
  - muscular dystrophy (e.g. myotonic dystrophy).

2. What particular aspects of the clinical examination might help narrow the differential diagnosis?

In any patient with dysarthria, the following should be performed:

- ◆ examination of the tongue for wasting and fasciculations
- ◆ examination for fatiguability, e.g. inability to sustain upgaze, or weakness of shoulder muscles when tested after repeated shoulder abduction.

Patients may complain of sudden-onset symptoms in MND or myasthenia. It is likely that the onset is not in fact 'sudden', but that the patients were initially unaware of a problem. Uncertainty as to the time course of symptom onset may be a particular problem in MND with associated frontotemporal dementia. In bulbar-onset MND, symptoms and signs may be absent outside the bulbar muscles, making the diagnosis more difficult—hence the importance of examining the tongue. Similarly, myasthenia may be restricted to the bulbar muscles with an absence of symptoms elsewhere. A high index of suspicion is required in order not to miss these disorders which are not infrequently referred to TIA clinics.

Further reading

Becker A, Hardmeier M, Steck AJ, Czaplinski A (2007). Primary lateral sclerosis presenting with isolated progressive pseudobulbar syndrome. *Eur J Neurol*; **14**: e3.

Hopkins LC (1994). Clinical features of myasthenia gravis. *Neurol Clin*; **12**: 243–61.

Klenner-Fisman G, Kott HS (1998). Myaesthenia gravis mimicking stroke in elderly patients. *Mayo Clinic Proc*; **73**: 1077–8.

Kluin KJ, Bromberg MB, Feldmann EL, *et al.* (1996). Dysphagia in elderly men with myasthenia gravis. *J Neurol Sci*; **138**: 49–52.

Santens P, Van Borsel J, Foncke E, *et al.* (1999). Progressive dysarthria. Case reports and a review of the literature. *Dement Geriatr Cogn Disord*; **10**: 231–6.

Vincent A, Clover L, Buckley C, *et al.* (2003). Evidence of underdiagnosis of myasthenia gravis in older people. *J Neurol Neurosurg Psychiatry*; **74** 1105–8.

Volanti P, Mannino M, Piccoli T, La Bella V (2007). Carcinoma of the tongue and bulbar-onset amyotrophic lateral sclerosis: unusual differential diagnosis. *Neurol Sci*; **28**: 151–3.

Case 28

A 65-year-old man was referred to the neurology clinic for assessment of his recurrent 'dizzy spells'. He described episodes of sudden-onset vertigo and nausea, which lasted between a few hours and some days. There were no other associated symptoms. He also had a history of migraine with aura, during which he developed slurred speech and word-finding difficulties, followed by a headache some hours later. The patient had had a single unprovoked generalized seizure 2 years earlier, but otherwise he had always been healthy. His brother had a stroke at the age of 49 years. Neurological examination was normal. The patient's MRI brain is shown in Fig. 28.1.

Questions

1. Describe the findings on the MRI (Fig. 28.1). What do they show?
2. What is the most likely diagnosis? What other diagnoses would you consider?
3. Describe the clinical features of this condition. Do you think that the patient's dizziness is relevant? If so, how?
4. Which further investigations would you do to confirm the diagnosis?
5. How would you manage this patient?

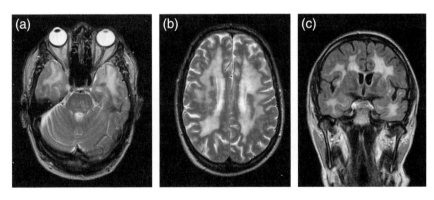

Fig. 28.1 MRI brain.

Answers

1. Describe the findings on the MRI (Fig. 28.1). What do they show?

Fig. 28.1(a) and (b) show axial T2-weighted images of the brain; Fig. 28.1(c) is a coronal FLAIR image. The images show widespread changes with high signal in the subcortical white matter, which also affect the temporal poles (Fig. 28.1(a) and (c)).

2. What is the most likely diagnosis? What other diagnoses would you consider?

The changes are consistent with cerebral small vessel disease. However, the patient is still quite young, and he does not have a history of hypertension. Therefore the changes appear too extensive to be explained by the small vessel changes that are usually found with increasing age and hypertension. Also, such changes would not usually affect the temporal lobes. The patient's history of migraine with aura and of a previous seizure, together with a family history of young-onset stroke suggests CADASIL (cerebral autosomal dominant arteriopathy with subcortical infarcts and leukoencephalopathy) as the most likely diagnosis. From the scan appearance, a leukodystrophy or perhaps advanced multiple sclerosis could also be considered, but the clinical history does not suggest these.

3. Describe the clinical features of this condition. Do you think that the patient's dizziness is relevant? If so, how?

CADASIL is an autosomal dominant vasculopathy that affects the small penetrating arteries of the brain, as well as leptomeningeal arteries and arterioles elsewhere in the body. The disease is due to a mutation in the *NOTCH* 3 gene on chromosome 19. This is a large gene with 33 exons, of which exons 3–6 are most commonly affected by mutations and are also the ones that will be screened first on genetic testing. The prominent clinical features of CADASIL are migraine with aura, young-onset strokes, cognitive decline, and psychiatric disturbances. These do not all have to be present. Frequently, there is a family history of early stroke, migraine, or dementia, or of other neurological illness, although new mutations also occur.

Symptoms usually develop in early adulthood, although they may not be obvious until the sixth decade. Migraine with aura is often the first clinical manifestation. It usually occurs between the ages of 20 and 40 years and will affect 40% of patients. Frequently, patients may have migraine with a complicated aura, for example, there is a high prevalence of hemiplegic migraine or basilar migraine. Although our patient's vertigo does not have any other migrainous features, 'migrainous vertigo', and 'vestibular migraine' are described entities. In the absence of any other explanation it appears likely that his attacks of vertigo are migrainous in origin. Ischaemic stroke is the most common clinical manifestation of CADASIL and will affect 85% of patients. Infarcts will usually be subcortical, and two-thirds are classical lacunar syndromes. Strokes or TIAs occur at a mean age of 45–50 years, but may occur as early as age 20 years and up to age 70 years. Cognitive decline and impairment are the second most common features of CADASIL, and executive function is the most commonly affected domain. The prevalence of dementia increases with increasing age, and 60% of CADASIL patients over the age of 60 years will be demented. Mood disturbance and psychiatric illness are further features of CADASIL, and affect up to 40% of patients. Depression and bipolar disorder have both been reported. Five to ten per cent of patients will develop seizures during the course of their illness. As the disease progresses, patients may also develop gait difficulties, incontinence, and pseudobulbar palsy. Death usually occurs from secondary complications, commonly pneumonia, at a mean age of 65 years.

4. Which further investigations would you do to confirm the diagnosis?

In this patient, the clinical history taken together with the imaging findings are highly suggestive of CADASIL. Further confirmation can be obtained from genetic testing. Usually exons 3–6, where mutations are most common, will be screened first. Skin biopsy is another means of testing for CADASIL. If positive, it will show granular osmiophilic material in the media of blood vessels on electron microscopy (Fig. 28.2). This method is very specific, but has a relatively low sensitivity of 40%.

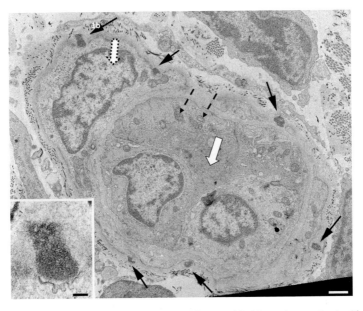

Fig. 28.2 Electron microscopy of a small vessel from a skin biopsy in a patient with CADASIL. The black arrows indicate the granular osmiophilic material in the blood vessel wall. The material is shown in more detail in the insert. For comparison, the black dashed arrows show the mitochondria, the white arrow shows the vessel lumen, and the white arrow with dashed lining shows the nucleus of a pericyte.

Immunostaining with anti-*NOTCH* 3 antibodies is an alternative to electron microscopy, but its specificity and sensitivity have yet to be determined.

5. How would you manage this patient?

There is no specific treatment for CADASIL; management is purely symptomatic. Migraine can be treated with migraine prophylactics. Some authors have suggested that acetazolamide is helpful in managing migraine. Patients are often given aspirin for stroke prevention. However, this is pragmatic, as the underlying disease process is different from that of stroke caused by atheromatous disease, and there is no evidence that aspirin prevents stroke in CADASIL. Dual antiplatelet therapy and anticoagulation should be avoided, as patients frequently have microhaemorrhages and there may be an increased risk of bleeding. Statins are frequently prescribed because of their assumed beneficial effect on endothelial dysfunction. Again, there is no evidence that they improve outcome in CADASIL. Seizures usually respond well to anticonvulsants, and psychiatric symptoms should be managed appropriately (e.g. with serotonin re-uptake inhibitors). In the long term, physiotherapy, management of incontinence, and nasogastric/percutaneous endoscopic gastroscopy (PEG) feeding will be required.

Our patient is currently still very well, and apart from migraine treatment does not require any specific management. However, he has two sons. One of the sons has a history of migraine with aura, and he has also been diagnosed with 'chronic fatigue syndrome'. There is a suspicion that he may also be affected by CADASIL, and the family are currently undergoing genetic counselling. This is also a very important aspect of the management of patients with CADASIL and their families. CADASIL usually presents at an age when the patients already have children. The penetrance of the disease is high, it is relentlessly progressive, and no treatment is available. Within this context, a patient and his family will require ongoing support and counselling, and genetic testing of relatives will have to be considered carefully.

Further reading

Razvi SM, Muir KW (2004). Cerebral autosomal dominant arteriopathy with subcortical infarcts and leukoencephalopathy. *Pract Neurol*; **4**: 50–5.

Tournier-Lasserve E, Joutel A, Melki J, *et al.* (1993). Cerebral autosomal dominant arteriopathy with subcortical infarcts and leukoencephalopathy maps to chromosome 19q12. *Nat Genet*; **3**: 256–9.

Case 29

Case 29.A

A 59-year-old man was referred to the TIA clinic for a suspected brainstem stroke. While on a flight from Cape Town to London, he had suddenly noticed that he saw two 'exit' signs, one almost exactly above the other. There was no headache, vertigo, nausea, or any other focal neurological deficit. However, his symptoms of vertical diplopia persisted. Examination was entirely normal, except for reported vertical diplopia which was worst when looking straight ahead, although the eyes were parallel in this position with no obvious deviation. Eye movements were normal. The diplopia disappeared when the patient covered either eye.

Case 29.B

A 34-year-old woman was referred to the neurovascular clinic for urgent assessment of left partial ptosis initially noticed by her husband. She reported that symptoms had been present for about a month. The ptosis was worse in the evenings and when she was tired. She did not complain of diplopia or any other visual symptoms, but her husband reported that her left eye often appeared not to be looking in the same direction as her right eye. She was a non-smoker and had an unremarkable past medical history. She had lost approximately 10kg in weight over the past 6 months.

On examination, the left eyelid sat just below the start of the iris. Her pupils were equal in size and were reactive to light and accommodation. The conjunctivae were injected bilaterally and the eyes appeared prominent. There was a full range of eye movements with no diplopia elicited. There was no lid lag or fatiguability on sustained upgaze. The rest of the CN examination, limb examination, and reflexes were normal.

Questions

1. Where do you think the lesion is located in Case 29.A? Give reasons.

2. How would you assess patient A further?

3. What diagnosis do you think that the doctor who organized the urgent neurovascular referral had in mind as a potentially dangerous underlying condition in Case 29.B?

4. Give a differential diagnosis for patient B. What do you think the most likely diagnosis is?

5. List the eye signs that occur in association with the most likely diagnosis in Case 29.B.

Answers

1. Where do you think the lesion is located in Case 29.A? Give reasons.

To assess diplopia, it is first of all useful to determine if the patient has monocular or binocular diplopia. In monocular diplopia, double vision will persist as long as the patient keeps the affected eye open. Monocular diplopia is caused by conditions affecting the structure of the eye, for example dislocation of the lens. Binocular diplopia is only present when the patient has both eyes open, and it disappears when the patient covers either eye. Binocular diplopia is due to defects in the eye muscles, neuromuscular junction, oculomotor nerves, or supranuclear brainstem pathways. Although the patient described here has no obvious eye movement abnormality, this can often be subtle, and his binocular diplopia suggests a lesion distal to the eye.

2. How would you assess patient A further?

Further investigations should include a detailed orthoptic review to assess the presence and pattern of any eye movement abnormalities. Depending on these findings, further investigations would include imaging of the orbits and eye muscles to look for structural lesions that inhibit eye movements or signal change in the eye muscles, for example suggestive of myositis or infiltration. Brain imaging, preferably with MRI, might reveal a compressive lesion of a CN, or a lesion in the midbrain. Acetylcholine receptor antibodies to check for myasthenia gravis should also be done, as should thyroid function tests, anti-microsomal antibodies, and anti-thyroglobulin antibodies to assess for Graves' disease.

All of these investigations were normal in patient A. Further ophthalmological assessment revealed that he had 'macular wrinkling'. This is a condition in which the internal limiting membrane of the eye is deformed, usually due to traction at the vitreo-retinal interface. This may occur in diabetic retinopathy, in macular degeneration, or with chorio-retinal scarring. Usually symptoms consist of blurred vision or metamorphopsia, i.e. objects appear distorted. However, retinal wrinkling may sometimes result in displacement of the macula, and then the retinal images of a fixed object will not be on retinotopically corresponding points. In this case, patients may experience binocular diplopia, even though the lesion is located within the eye. In patient A, the assumption was that the changes in air pressure experienced during flying might have caused the macular wrinkling.

3. What diagnosis do you think that the doctor who organized the urgent neurovascular referral had in mind as a potentially dangerous underlying condition in Case 29.B?

The patient was referred with a suspected oculomotor (third) nerve palsy. This may be caused by compression of the third nerve by an aneurysm of the posterior communicating artery, which may cause SAH. While this is an important diagnosis to consider in patients who present with ptosis, it is unlikely in this case.

Third nerve palsies due to compression by a posterior communicating artery aneurysm usually present with a combination of the following:

◆ **Ptosis**, which may be complete or at least severe enough to cover the pupil.

◆ **Diplopia**: classically, the eye is positioned 'down and out' in a third nerve palsy, and patients complain of diagonal double vision. This may be absent if the ptosis is severe enough to impair vision out of the affected eye.

◆ **Anisocoria**: the pupil in the affected eye will be dilated. This is due to compression of the parasympathetic nerve fibres in the third nerve. These lie very superficially in the subarachnoid portion of the third nerve, and they are generally affected in the presence of an aneurysm. This is in contrast to a 'pupil-sparing third nerve palsy', which is usually due to an ischaemic nerve lesion, for example in diabetic patients. In these cases, the core of the nerve is affected, and the parasympathetic fibres are often spared—an important distinguishing feature to a compressive nerve lesion.

The patient described here has only an incomplete ptosis with no clear eye-movement abnormality and normal pupil size. Therefore it is very unlikely that she has a third nerve palsy.

4. Give a differential diagnosis for patient B. What do you think the most likely diagnosis is?

This patient has an incomplete ptosis, with some fatiguability. There may be a subtle eye movement abnormality. The patient has had significant weight loss, and on examination there are injected conjunctivae and perhaps a degree of proptosis.

The combination of weight loss and eye movement abnormalities makes hyperthyroidism with thyroid eye disease the main diagnosis to be considered. Thyroid function needs to be checked, as well as thyroid auto-antibodies (anti-thyroid peroxidase, anti-thyroglobulin, and thyroid-stimulating antibodies). Imaging of the orbits will be helpful. In thyroid eye disease, this will show enlargement of the ocular muscles in both orbits (Fig. 29.1). Treatment consists of treating the hyperthyroidism. They eye may require lubricant drops to protect it from corneal ulceration.

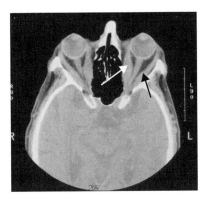

Fig. 29.1 Enlargement of ocular muscles in thyroid eye disease (arrows).

Steroids are often used for treatment, and surgery may be required in more severe cases.

A differential diagnosis in this patient would include myasthenia gravis, in particular because she mentioned some fatiguability in the severity of her ptosis. Anti-acetylcholine receptor antibodies should be checked, and if there are any other symptoms suggestive of myasthenia, neurophysiological studies may be helpful to confirm this diagnosis.

Other diagnoses to be considered in this patient include orbital tumours or inflammatory lesions, although these would rarely be bilateral. In patients with a red prominent eye, a carotico-cavernous fistula should always be considered, but this is usually unilateral. There is often pulsatile tinnitus. In this patient, the combination of weight loss, bilateral symptoms, and eye movement abnormalities made thyroid eye disease the most likely diagnosis. This was confirmed by thyroid function tests and imaging.

5. List the eye signs that occur in association with the most likely diagnosis in Case 29.B.

Eye signs that occur in thyroid eye disease include the following:

- ◆ Chemosis (conjunctival oedema).
- ◆ Periorbital oedema.
- ◆ Exophthalmos—affects around 30–50% of patients.
- ◆ Proptosis (occasionally unilateral).
- ◆ Ophthalmoplegia due to lymphocytic infiltration of the eye muscles. This can cause diplopia and may lead to a complex ophthalmoplegia involving numerous ocular muscles.

Further reading

Barton JJS (2004). 'Retinal diplopia' associated with macular wrinkling. *Neurology*; **63**: 925–7.

Cawood T, Moriarty P, O'Shea D (2004). Recent developments in thyroid eye disease. *BMJ*; **329**: 385–90.

Case 30

A 50-year-old woman was referred to the TIA clinic by her GP. She had just returned from France where she had been hospitalized 2 months previously with an intracerebral bleed affecting the thalamus and left temporal lobe. She had made a good recovery but was left with a right lower quadrant visual field defect and reduced sensation in the right face, arm, and leg. She had been diagnosed as hypertensive 6 months prior to her stroke but otherwise had been well. Investigations in France, which had consisted of brain imaging (CT and MRI) and blood tests, including vasculitis screen, had shown no cause other than hypertension and a diagnosis of primary intracerebral bleed secondary to hypertension had been made.

At the TIA clinic in the UK, general systems examination was unremarkable and neurological findings were as documented previously in France.

Repeat screening bloods, including clotting, inflammatory markers, and auto-antibodies, were normal.

Questions—Part 1

1. List the causes of spontaneous intracranial haemorrhage. What are the most likely causes of this woman's intracerebral haemorrhage?
2. How would you manage this patient?

Answers

1. List the causes of spontaneous intracranial haemorrhage. What are the most likely causes of this woman's intracerebral haemorrhage?

The causes of spontaneous intracranial haemorrhage are shown in Table 30.1.

Table 30.1 Causes of spontaneous intracranial haemorrhage

Hypertension
Cerebral amyloid angiopathy (see Case 6)
Intracranial vascular malformations
arteriovenous,
venous, cavernous (see Case 44)
telangiectasis
Tumours (see Case 1)
secondary (melanoma, hypernephroma, endometrial carcinoma, bronchogenic carcinoma, choriocarcinoma)
primary
Haemostatic failure
haemophilia and other coagulation disorders
anticoagulation
thrombolysis (see Case 51)
antiplatelet drugs
disseminated intravascular coagulation
thrombocytopenia
thrombotic thrombocytopenic purpura
polycythaemia rubra vera
essential thrombocythaemia
paraproteinaemias
renal failure
liver failure
snake bite
Aneurysms
saccular (see Case 21)
atheromatous
mycotic
myxomatous
dissecting
Inflammatory vascular disease

Table 30.1 (Continued) Causes of spontaneous intracranial haemorrhage

Haemorrhagic transformation of cerebral infarction, venous more often than arterial (see Fig. 30.1)

Intracranial venous thrombosis (see Case 17)

Recreational drugs

Infections

 infective endocarditis (IE) (see Case 47)

 herpes simplex

 leptospirosis

 anthrax

Sickle-cell disease

Moyamoya syndrome (see Case 40)

Carotid endarterectomy (see Cases 19 and 32)

Intracranial surgery

Alcohol

Wernicke's encephalopathy

Chronic meningitis

Occult trauma

Reversible cerebral vasoconstriction (see Case 34)

The most likely causes of this woman's ICH are:

- primary ICH secondary to hypertension
- space-occupying lesion
- vascular malformation.

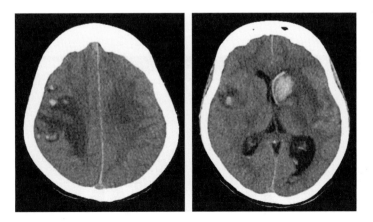

Fig. 30.1 Haemorrhagic transformation of infarct. This patient had multiple cardioembolic infarcts. There is a petechial haemorrhagic transformation in the right MCA territory, and more significant haemorrhagic transformation of a left-sided caudate nucleus infarct.

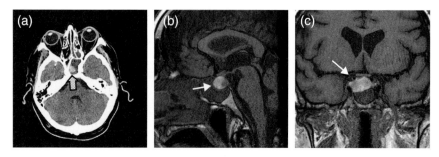

Fig. 30.2 Brain imaging from a patient who complained of headache and double vision after receiving thrombolysis for a myocardial infarction. Axial CT brain slice (a) shows a mass lesion centred on an expanded pituitary fossa with some destruction of bone on the right. A portion of the lesion is hyperdense, consistent with recent haemorrhage (arrow). Sagittal (b) and coronal (c) T1-weighted MRI confirms an intrasellar mass lesion extending into the right cavernous sinus and medial cerebral fossa (arrows). The lesion extends upwards and is in contact with the optic chiasm which, however, is not compressed or displaced. The appearances are consistent with a pituitary adenoma.

It is often difficult to establish the underlying cause of a spontaneous intracranial haemorrhage. The site of bleeding may give some information since the relative frequency of the various pathologies causing intracranial haemorrhage varies by site (see Case 6). However, most parts of the brain may be affected by any of the causes listed in Table 30.1. Occasionally, use of anticoagulation or thrombolysis may reveal a tumour through precipitation of haemorrhage (Fig. 30.2).

The most common cause of primary ICH is intracranial small vessel disease associated with hypertension followed by CAA (see Case 6) and intracranial vascular malformations. Hypertensive haemorrhages (see Fig. 30.3) tend to occur in the basal ganglia, thalamus, and pons, while lobar haemorrhages are more often due to CAA, vascular malformations, and haemostatic failure.

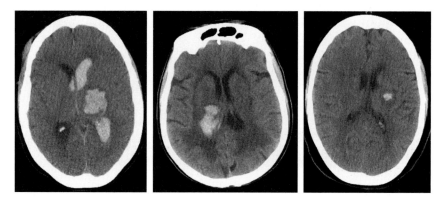

Fig. 30.3 Examples of hypertensive basal ganglia haemorrhages.

The current patient was known to be hypertensive and the site of haemorrhage was around the thalamus, and thus the diagnosis of hypertensive haemorrhage would seem reasonable. However, it is rare for patients under 55 to present with hypertensive bleeds; the incidence of primary ICH rises exponentially with age. Therefore other possible causes should be considered, including vascular malformations (although these more often cause lobar bleeding) and neoplastic lesions. Haemostatic mechanisms and infective and inflammatory causes were felt to be unlikely in this patient in view of the normal investigation results and the fact that she remained systemically well. CAA would not be expected to cause thalamic bleeding and, except for rare familial forms, is a disease of the elderly (see Case 6).

2. How would you manage this patient?

Management includes aggressive antihypertensive therapy and further brain imaging.

Where there is uncertainty as to the underlying cause of ICH, as in the current case, patients should be followed up not just to ensure adherence to secondary preventive measures, but also to ensure that the initial diagnosis is correct and that the clinical course proceeds as expected. It is not uncommon for the diagnosis to be revised on the basis of subsequent clinical developments (see Case 1) or further investigation results. This patient should be referred for repeat brain MRI and possibly formal angiography depending on the outcome of patient and physician discussion regarding risks and benefits.

Case progression

At the initial consultation, the TIA clinic physician decided that, in view of the patient's young age and previously mild hypertension only, the cause of the stroke was uncertain. An underlying vascular abnormality or structural lesion could not be excluded. She therefore arranged for a repeat MRI brain with GRE sequences to look for evidence of microbleeds (see Cases 2, 6, and 41). The presence of microbleeds would make the diagnosis of hypertensive haemorrhage more likely. The patient declined formal angiography at this point after discussion of the risks (which were difficult to predict in a young patient with uncertain pathology).

One week later, before repeat MRI was performed, the patient had a further ICH, again centred on the thalamus. Brain imaging showed blood, but no underlying abnormality was visible. She made a reasonable recovery and agreed to formal angiography scheduled for 6 weeks later when recovery was sufficient to allow a definitive study. Unfortunately, the patient suffered a catastrophic intracerebral bleed and died before further investigations could be performed.

Questions—Part 2

3. What are the causes of recurrent intracerebral bleeding?

4. What is the most likely cause of the recurrent intracerebral bleeding in this case?

Answers

3. What are the causes of recurrent intracerebral bleeding?

The causes of recurrent intracerebral bleeding are shown in Table 30.2.

In general, the causes of intracerebral bleeding will vary according to whether the bleeding recurs at the same site or at a different site and the age of the patient. In this case, recurrent bleeding into the same brain region strongly suggests the presence of an underlying abnormality such as a tumour or AV malformation. Figure 30.4 shows a bleeding AV malformation.

Table 30.2 Causes of multiple spontaneous intracerebral haemorrhages

CAA (see Case 6)
Tumour (primary or secondary) (see Case 1)
Haemostatic defect
Thrombolytic drugs (see Case 51)
Multiple haemorrhagic infarcts (usually embolic from the heart) (see Case 47 and Fig. 30.1)
Intracranial venous thrombosis (see Case 17)
Inflammatory vascular disease (see Cases 11 and 25)
Intracranial vascular malformations (see Case 44 and Fig. 30.4)
Malignant hypertension
Eclampsia
Recreational drug use

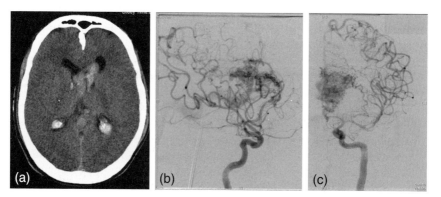

Fig. 30.4 Patient with an intraventricular haemorrhage ((a) CT brain) due to a large AV malformation arising from the left anterior cerebral artery ((b), (c) intra-arterial angiogram).

4. What is the most likely cause of the recurrent intracerebral bleeding in this case?

The most likely cause of the recurrent haemorrhages in this case is a tumour. Imaging of another patient with a similar presentation is shown in Fig. 30.5.

Most of the causes of recurrent spontaneous intracerebral bleeding listed in Table 30.2 result in bleeds separated in both space and time. Repeated bleeds at the same site make an underlying structural abnormality likely. Post-mortem examination on this patient revealed an aggressive glioblastoma originating in the thalamus.

This case illustrates the importance of follow-up and reconsideration of the initial diagnosis in patients with apparent stroke (see also Case 1).

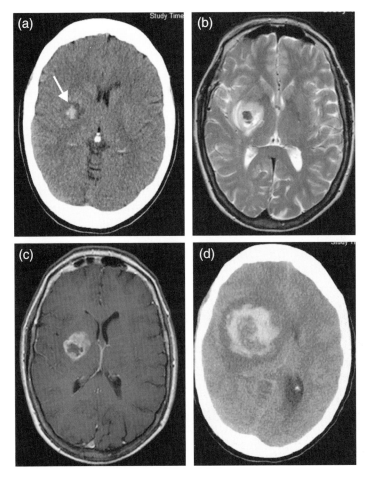

Fig. 30.5 CT brain (a) of a patient presenting with a small right basal ganglia haemorrhage (arrow). MRI brain showed a haemorrhagic core with perilesional oedema (b), but also avid enhancement on T1-weighted imaging with Gadolinium (c), which appeared more than expected for a haemorrhage and raised suspicion of an underlying tumour. The patient had a further haemorrhage into the tumour (d), and was eventually diagnosed as having a glioblastoma.

Further reading

Dickinson CJ (2001). Why are strokes related to hypertension? Classic studies and hypotheses revisited. *J Hypertens*; **19**: 1515–21.

Smith EE, Eichler F (2006). Cerebral amyloid angiopathy and lobar intracerebral hemorrhage. *Arch Neurol*; **63**: 148–51.

Stapf C, Mast H, Sciacca RR, *et al.* (2006). Predictors of hemorrhage in patients with untreated brain arteriovenous malformation. *Neurology*; **66**: 1350–5.

Sutherland GR, Auer RN (2006). Primary intracerebral hemorrhage. *J Clin Neurosci*; **13**: 511–17.

van Beijnum J, Lovelock CE, Cordonnier C, *et al.* (2009). Outcome after spontaneous and arteriovenous malformation-related intracerebral haemorrhage: population-based studies. *Brain*; **132**: 537–43.

Case 31

A 75-year-old woman, who was previously well, presented with a sudden-onset severe left-sided headache, which she likened to being hit with a brick. This was associated with non-specific dizziness, a tingling sensation in the left hand and the left side of the face, and a slight left facial droop. Symptoms were severe for 10 minutes, after which the patient was left with a generalized moderately severe headache and feeling 'woozy'. On admission to the emergency department, her blood pressure was 210/90mmHg. She had no focal neurological deficit. She was investigated for a possible SAH. A CT brain scan was normal, but the subsequent lumbar puncture was unhelpful because of a traumatic tap. A CT angiogram showed a possible aneurysm of the right ICA, and an intra-arterial angiogram was arranged for further investigation. The angiogram confirmed a 2mm ectasia of the carotid artery in the siphon which was of no therapeutic consequence. It also showed widespread segmental stenoses involving all the vascular territories in the major intracranial arteries as well as the distal more peripheral branches (Fig. 31.1) A subsequent MRI brain scan and MRA two days later confirmed these findings and also showed multiple small infarcts in all vascular territories, some microhaemorrhages, and moderate small vessel disease (Figs 31.2 and 31.3). The patient remained in hospital while she was investigated. Her headache settled over a few days, and there was no recurrence of her severe initial headache. She developed no neurological deficit. Her blood pressure proved difficult to control, but was around 150/90mmHg on discharge, following treatment with amlodipine and a thiazide diuretic.

Questions

1. Taking into account the clinical history and imaging findings, what is your differential diagnosis?
2. How would you investigate this patient further?
3. How would you treat this patient?

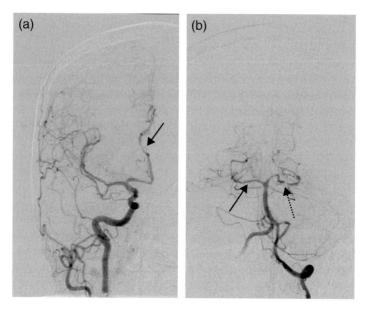

Fig. 31.1 Intra-arterial angiogram: (a) right common carotid artery injection; (b) left vertebral artery injection. The arrows show narrowing in the right anterior cerebral artery (a), and in both posterior cerebral arteries (b), with multiple short stenoses and beading on the right (solid arrow) and a more severe short segment stenosis on the left (dashed arrow).

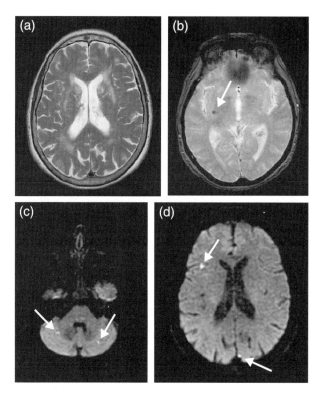

Fig. 31.2 MRI brain scan. The T2-weighted image shows diffuse periventricular white matter disease (a). GRE (b) shows a microhaemorrhage in the right putamen. Diffusion-weighted imaging shows small acute infarcts in both cerebellar hemispheres (c) and in the left occipital cortex and right frontal cortex (d).

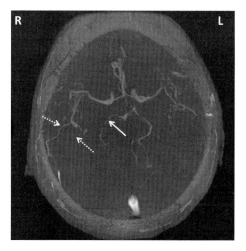

Fig 31.3 MRA. This shows diffuse widespread narrowing of the cerebral vessels. In particular, the beadlike appearance of the right posterior cerebral artery shown in Figure 31.1 is also visible here (solid arrow). There are also multiple stenoses of the more distal branches of the right middle cerebral artery (dashed arrows).

Answers

1. Taking into account the clinical history and imaging findings, what is your differential diagnosis?

Clinically this woman presented with 'thunderclap headache' and newly diagnosed hypertension. A SAH was not confirmed, but she was found to have widespread segmental stenoses of the intracranial arteries, and her MRI scan showed small vessel disease, microhaemorrhages, and multiple small acute infarcts.

Multiple stenoses on vascular imaging could be due to vasospasm, vasculitis, or intracranial atheroma, but the clinical presentation is not consistent with all of these.

Vasospasm can occur after a SAH. Although this woman presented with a thunderclap headache, we found no evidence of subarachnoid blood, and no source for a SAH on vascular imaging. Vasospasm can also occur in RCVS or Call–Fleming syndrome (see also Case 34). In this syndrome, patients present with thunderclap headache, which is usually recurrent, and vascular imaging shows widespread stenoses. Typically, patients are younger than our patient, with a mean age of onset of 45 years. There is a provoking factor (e.g. exposure to vasoactive substances or being post-partum) in 60% of patients. Hypertension has also been suggested as a risk factor for RCVS. Patients with RCVS may develop seizures, and haemorrhagic or ischaemic strokes. Cerebral infarctions are usually in a posterior location in the watershed territory. RCVS, perhaps provoked by hypertension, appeared a possible diagnosis in our patient, although her infarct pattern was different from that usually described, she had had only one episode of thunderclap headache, and she was also unusually old for this diagnosis.

Cerebral vasculitis of the medium-sized intracranial vessels was high on the list of differential diagnoses, given the vascular imaging appearances. The combination of white matter changes, multiple ischaemic infarctions, and microhaemorrhages would also have been in keeping with a diagnosis of small vessel vasculitis. However, the clinical presentation would have been atypical. Usually cerebral vasculitis has a slower insidious onset. Patients may have a headache, but this is milder, generalized, and not sudden onset. Patients are often generally unwell, whereas our patient was systemically very well. Further investigations should include a search for systemic markers of vasculitis, a CSF examination, and potentially a brain biopsy.

Intracranial atheroma is a further diagnosis to be considered in this patient. This is generally thought to be more common in Afro-Caribbean and Asian populations, but more recently has also been described with increasing frequency in Caucasians. Intracranial atheromatous disease is now thought to account for 5–10% of ischaemic strokes. No specific risk factors for intracranial atheroma have yet been identified, but hypertension is certainly a risk factor. Our patient had white matter disease and microhaemorrhages on brain imaging. These changes would be in keeping with hypertensive small vessel disease. It transpired that she had not seen her family physician for years, so her hypertension may well have gone unnoticed for a long time. Long-standing hypertension would also account for intracranial atheroma and, given that she was otherwise well, this was felt to be the most likely diagnosis.

2. How would you investigate this patient further?

The possibility of cerebral vasculitis had to be investigated further in this woman, as this is a treatable condition with possibly devastating consequences. Her inflammatory markers were normal and auto-antibodies, including antinuclear factor (ANF) and antineutrophil cytoplasmic antibody (ANCA), were negative. Repeat CSF examination 3 days after symptom onset was entirely normal. This would be highly unusual in cerebral vasculitis, which shows abnormal CSF in more than 95% of cases. The next step would have been to proceed to brain biopsy to look for inflammatory changes. However, this carries a procedural risk and, given that our patient was well, we felt that a diagnosis of vasculitis was sufficiently unlikely to adopt a conservative approach at this stage.

The patient presented with new-onset hypertension, although in retrospect that may have been longer-standing. Nevertheless, episodes of hypertension and thunderclap headache have been described in phaeochromocytoma. In our patient, urinary catecholamines were normal. Abdominal ultrasound, which also looked for a renal artery stenosis, was also normal. There was left ventricular hypertrophy on echocardiogram, suggesting that the hypertension was not new.

In addition to investigating the hypertension, the patient should also be investigated for other vascular risk factors, given the potential diagnosis of intracranial atheroma. Hypercholesterolaemia is a risk factor for intracranial disease, and this woman's cholesterol level was 7mmol/L. She was not diabetic, but there was a remote smoking history until the age of 50 years. The patient also had an echocardiogram, which did not show a cardioembolic source for her multiple small infarcts.

RCVS is diagnosed by repeat vascular imaging 1–3 months after symptom onset. The patient had a further MRI brain and MRA of her intracranial vessels 3 months later. This showed no change in the appearance of the blood vessels. There were no new haemorrhages or infarctions. Overall, after this repeat imaging study and further review of the patient, who continued to do well, the most likely diagnosis for the appearance of her intracranial vasculature was widespread intracranial atheroma. The white matter changes and microhaemorrhages were felt to be in keeping with hypertensive small vessel disease. A possible explanation for the multiple small infarcts was that these were due to embolization during the intra-arterial angiography, which had been done 2 days prior to the original MRI scan.

3. How would you treat this patient?

The main initial consideration in this patient was whether to treat for a presumptive diagnosis of cerebral vasculitis. Such treatment would have consisted of high-dose steroids and further immunosuppressants, which clearly could have caused quite marked side effects. As the diagnosis of vasculitis seemed increasingly unlikely, we decided against immunosuppressive therapy. RCVS was a diagnosis we initially considered quite strongly. This syndrome usually improves spontaneously, but some studies report improvement with Ca antagonists (e.g. nimodipine). While it is uncertain whether these drugs do improve the outcome of RCVS, Ca antagonists are also used in the treatment of hypertension. Our patient required antihypertensive therapy, and we started her on a Ca antagonist in the hope that this would also be useful for any potential vasospasm. Her hypercholesterolaemia required treatment in its own right and, given the evidence of cerebral small vessel disease, we also felt it appropriate to start the patient on an antiplatelet agent.

In the end the most likely diagnosis in this patient was intracranial atheroma, although it remains uncertain if and how her original presentation with a thunder-clap headache was associated with this finding. We are treating the patient with a standard secondary stroke prevention regimen, and are monitoring her blood pressure closely. Endovascular treatment with angioplasty, and potentially stenting, is now available for intracranial atheroma, but it is not yet widely used and its benefit is still uncertain. Our patient had no single clearly symptomatic or particularly severe stenosis, and so endovascular treatment was not considered for her. Previously, patients with intracranial atheroma were often anticoagulated rather than given antiplatelet agents for stroke prevention. However, the WASID trial showed that warfarin had no clear benefit over aspirin, and that it caused more haemorrhages. Anticoagulation is no longer recommended for intracranial atheroma. Given our patient's microhaemorrhages, anticoagulation would have appeared risky, and we gave her aspirin.

Further reading

Caplan LR (2008). Intracranial large artery occlusive disease. *Curr Neurol Neurosci Rep*; **8**: 177–81.

Chimowitz MI, Lynn MJ, Howlett-Smith H, *et al.* (2005). Comparison of warfarin and aspirin for symptomatic intracranial arterial stenosis. *New Engl J Med*; **352**: 1305–16.

Ducros A, Bousser M-G (2009). Reversible cerebral vasoconstriction syndrome. *Pract Neurol*; **9**: 256–67

Küker W (2007). Cerebral vasculitis: imaging signs revisited. *Neuroradiology*; **49**: 471–9.

Taylor RA, Qureshi AI (2009). Intracranial atherosclerotic disease. *Curr Treat Options Neurol*; **11**: 444–51.

Case 32

A 78-year-old man developed sudden left arm weakness and dysarthria lasting for an hour and resolving spontaneously. The following day, he developed severe left arm weakness, left leg weakness, dysarthria, and left facial numbness. There was a past medical history of myocardial infarction, hypertension, and type 2 diabetes mellitus. He underwent diffusion-weighted MRI of the brain (Fig. 32.1).

Questions

1. Describe the mechanism of diffusion-weighted MRI. Why is it useful in the management of acute stroke and TIA?

2. What does the diffusion-weighted MRI from this case show? What is the most likely underlying cause?

3. How would you manage this patient?

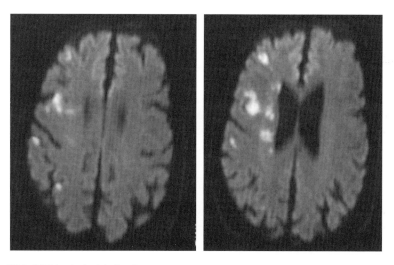

Fig. 32.1 DWI brain (axial slices).

Answers

1. Describe the mechanism of diffusion-weighted MRI. Why is it useful in the management of acute stroke and TIA?

DWI relies on changes in the Brownian motion of water molecules to generate contrast. During early ischaemia, cytotoxic oedema develops and water moves into the cells. Intracellular water movement is more restricted because of the presence of organelles and membranes. In addition, owing to cell swelling, the extracellular compartment reduces in size, so that water diffusion is also restricted here. Reduced proton diffusion leads to a high-signal (bright) DWI lesion. DWI has a high sensitivity for acute ischaemic stroke at around 90%, although it is not entirely specific for ischaemia, and other conditions such as seizure, encephalitis, and multiple sclerosis can all cause DWI lesions. Inter-observer agreement is better for DWI than with conventional MRI but there appears to be a lower sensitivity for DWI in posterior circulation acute stroke (19–31% false negatives), particularly where lesions are small and within the first 24 hours after stroke onset. While DWI makes recent ischaemic lesions easily visible, it is prone to 'T2 shine through', i.e. sometimes high-signal lesions on DWI may not be acute but secondary to high-signal lesions on T2-weighted imaging. To verify the acuity of a lesion on DWI, an ADC map is used. This is a map of the apparent diffusion coefficient, which purely shows diffusion and is not prone to any shine through effects. Areas with reduced diffusion have low signal; areas with high water mobility (e.g. CSF in the ventricles) show high signal. The low signal of a recent ischamic lesion on the ADC map is not easy to detect, which is why clinically the DWI is looked at first, and the acuity of any lesion then double-checked on the ADC map afterwards. The value of the ADC changes with time after stroke. It is reduced for the first 10–14 days after stroke onset. It then rises, may transiently become normal (pseudo-normalization), and will be high in a chronic infarct. The main advantage of DWI and of ADC mapping is that it allows us to distinguish between acute and chronic infarction, which is often not possible on conventional structural MRI.

The high sensitivity of DWI in acute stroke and its ability to distinguish between acute and chronic infarction make it useful in the management of acute stroke and TIA for the following reasons:

♦ DWI can help to confirm the diagnosis of a cerebral ischaemic event when the clinical history is uncertain.

♦ DWI helps to identify the presence of acute ischaemic lesions which may not be identifiable on T2-weighted imaging, for example in the presence of diffuse white matter disease or brain atrophy (Fig. 32.2).

♦ DWI can help to determine the vascular territory affected by an infarct, for example whether the anterior or the posterior circulation is affected (Fig. 32.3). This is often not possible using clinical criteria alone.

♦ DWI can be helpful in establishing stroke aetiology. For example, the demonstration of multiple acute lesions affecting both hemispheres would suggest a cardioembolic cause (see Case 4), vasculitis (see Cases 11 and 25), or IVBCL (see Case 50).

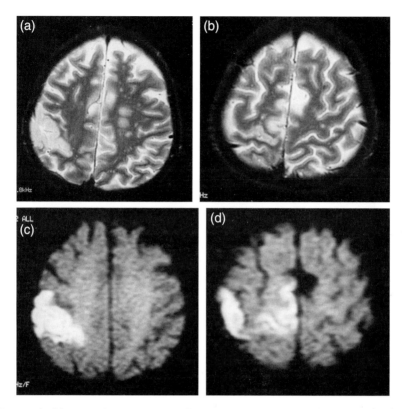

Fig. 32.2 (a, b) T2-weighted images and (c, d) DWI of a patient presenting with an acute right MCA stroke. While the wedge-shaped infarct in the posterior MCA-territory is visible on both T2 (a) and DWI (c), the acute infarct affecting the medial right hemisphere is much more clearly visible on DWI (d) than on T2 (b) because of brain atrophy and the presence of high signal from the CSF, which makes it difficult to identify infarcted cortical tissue on this imaging sequence.

♦ The combination of DWI with perfusion-weighted imaging to measure cerebral blood flow can sometimes influence patient selection for thrombolysis beyond the current 3 hour (some centres use 4.5 hours) treatment window through the demonstration of potentially salvageable ischaemic tissue (the ischaemic penumbra) (see below).

2. What does the diffusion-weighted MRI from this case show? What is the most likely underlying cause?

The diffusion-weighted MRI from this patient (Fig. 32.1) shows multiple acute infarcts within the anterior circulation of the right hemisphere. The presence of multiple infarcts in one hemisphere suggests embolization from the ipsilateral carotid artery. Most commonly, this will be due to an atheromatous carotid stenosis, although it

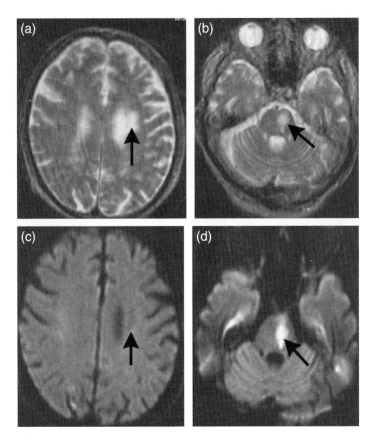

Fig. 32.3 (a,b) T2-weighted MRI (a,b) and (c, d) DWI of a patient who presented with an acute right hemiparesis. The T2-weighted images (a,b) show a left subcortical (a) and a left pontine (b) infarct, but it is not possible to say which infarct is acute. DWI shows low signal for the subcortical infarct, and confirms the pontine infarct as acute (d). This clarifies that the patient has had an acute ischaemic event affecting the posterior circulation.

may also occur after a carotid dissection with thrombus developing on an intimal flap (see Fig. 32.4).

3. How would you manage this patient?

The scan appearance strongly suggests the presence of carotid disease, and therefore urgent carotid imaging is required. If this confirms the presence of a severe carotid stenosis, the patient should be considered for urgent carotid endarterctomy, as this reduces the risk of subsequent stroke (see Case 19). Medical secondary prevention therapy with antiplatelet agents, statins, and blood-pressure lowering should be started as soon as possible. The treatment of carotid dissection is discussed in Case 24.

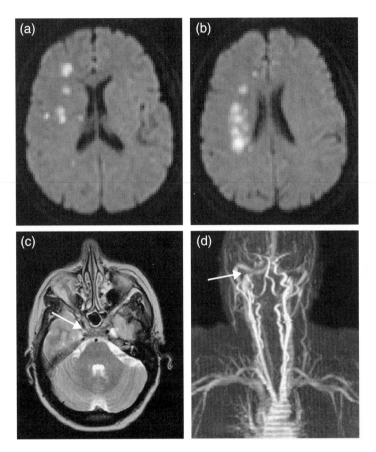

Fig. 32.4 MR images from a young patient with a right carotid dissection. DWI ((a) and (b)) shows multiple acute infarcts in the right hemisphere, axial T2-weighted MRI (c) shows a dissected right carotid with an intimal flap (arrow), and TOF-MRA (d) shows an occluded right carotid artery after dissection. (arrow, compare to contralateral left ICA which is clearly visible).

This patient received medical secondary preventive therapy and went on to have a carotid endarterectomy for his 80% carotid stenosis, from which he made an uneventful recovery.

Further reading

Schulz UG, Briley D, Meagher T, Molyneux A, Rothwell PM (2003). Abnormalities on diffusion weighted magnetic resonance imaging performed several weeks after a minor stroke or transient ischaemic attack. *J Neurol Neurosurg Psychiatry*; **74**: 734–8.

Schulz UG, Briley D, Meagher T, Molyneux A, Rothwell PM (2004). Diffusion-weighted MRI in 300 patients presenting late with subacute transient ischemic attack or minor stroke. *Stroke*; **35**: 2459–65.

Case 33

A 65-year-old man presented to the TIA clinic with a history of sudden-onset dysarthria and unsteadiness. He insisted that he had been completely well until then. However, his wife reported that over the past month he had been more irritable and forgetful, and that he had also had several falls. The patient's MRI scan is shown in Fig. 33.1.

Over the next few months the patient deteriorated rapidly. He developed myoclonic jerks, became increasingly unsteady and mute, and was eventually bedbound. He died 5 months after his original presentation to the TIA clinic.

Questions

1. Describe the findings on the MRI brain.
2. What is the diagnosis?
3. What other investigations would you do to confirm this diagnosis?

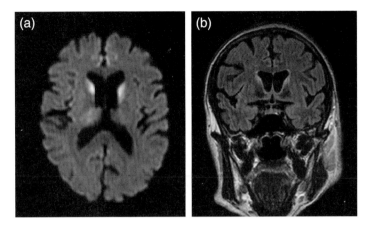

Fig. 33.1 MRI brain. Axial DWI (a) and coronal FLAIR (b).

Answers

1. Describe the findings on the MRI brain.

Figure 33.1(a) shows an axial diffusion-weighted image and Fig. 33.1(b) shows a coronal FLAIR sequence. The images show some brain atrophy, but the most striking change is the bilateral high signal in the caudate nucleus on both images.

2. What is the diagnosis?

Rapid cognitive decline, ataxia, myoclonus, and akinetic mutism in an elderly patient are a typical presentation of sporadic CJD. This is the most common form of human prion disease and occurs in about one per one million people per year. The disease is invariably fatal, usually within 5 months of symptom onset. There is no known effective treatment.

This patient deteriorated too rapidly for any of the common dementing illnesses (e.g. AD). Bilateral high signal in the caudate nucleus on several MRI sequences, including T2-weighted images, FLAIR, DWI, and proton-density weighted images is found in 70–80% of cases of sporadic CJD. High signal is also typically seen in the putamen, and sometimes other grey matter nuclei such as the pallidum, the peri-aqueductal grey matter, and the thalamus are affected. On DWI, there may already be diffusely high signal of the cortex in the early stages of the disease. Bilateral high signal in the basal ganglia on MRI may also be found in other diseases (e.g. Wilson's disease, mitochondrial disorders, encephalitis, Huntington's disease, or bilateral basal ganglia infarction). However, in the current case the imaging findings together with the clinical presentation are highly suggestive of a diagnosis of sporadic CJD. Even the rapid stroke-like onset of symptoms in CJD has been reported before and may occur in up to 20% of patients.

3. What other investigations would you do to confirm this diagnosis?

Further investigations to confirm a diagnosis of CJD should include CSF examination and EEG. Other investigations should be done according to the suspected differential diagnosis. In CJD, CSF may show a slightly raised protein, but its constituents are otherwise normal. CSF should be checked for levels of protein 14-3-3. These are usually raised in CJD, although they are only a marker of general neuronal breakdown and are not specific. EEG typically shows periodic triphasic sharp wave complexes. However, these may be absent early in the disease. Repeated EEGs may be helpful in establishing the diagnosis, as there will often be rapidly progressive changes over time, and about 60–80% of patients will eventually develop typical EEG changes during the course of the disease. A definite diagnosis of sporadic CJD can only be made by tissue diagnosis, usually post-mortem. A brain biopsy ante-mortem is not generally recommended and should only be done to diagnose a potentially treatable alternative disorder. It carries risks, the diagnosis of CJD may be missed as the disease distribution may be patchy, and the neurosurgical instruments would have to be destroyed after the procedure. Currently, therefore, the ante-mortem diagnosis of sporadic CJD is clinical. The diagnostic criteria have recently been revised as follows.

♦ Clinical presentation:
  - dementia
  - visual or cerebellar dysfunction
  - Pyramidal or extrapyramidal dysfunction
  - akinetic mutism.

♦ Additional investigation results:
  - periodic sharp wave complexes on EEG
  - protein 14-3-3 detected in the CSF
  - high-signal abnormalities in caudate nucleus, putamen, or at least two cortical regions on DWI or FLAIR.

A diagnosis of 'probable CJD' is made if at least two of the clinical and one of the investigation criteria apply. The criteria have 98% sensitivity and 71% specificity.

Further reading

Collie D (2002). Creutzfeld-Jakob disease. *Pract Neurol*; 2: 168–72.

Collins SJ, Lawson VA, Masters CL (2004). Transmissible spongiform encephalopathies. *Lancet*; 363: 51–61.

Zerr I, Kallenberg K, Summers DM, *et al.* (2009). Updated clinical diagnostic criteria for sporadic Creutzfeldt–Jakob disease. *Brain*; 132: 2659–68.

Case 34

A 43-year-old woman presented 10 days after a sudden-onset headache, which had persisted. Apart from the headache, she had no other symptoms and she looked clinically well. She was investigated for SAH. CT brain showed an area of hyperintense material in the cortical sulci at the vertex that was thought to be haemorrhage (Fig. 34.1). She proceeded to CTA which showed no aneurysm or arteriovenous malformation but did show irregularities of the distal posterior ICA bilaterally (Fig. 34.2). This unusual appearance led to a lumbar puncture (LP) being performed which was normal (no polymorphs, two lymphocytes, 640 red cells, no xanthochromia). MRI brain showed no brain lesion except for the area of hyperdense material in the cortical sulci at the vertex previously seen on CT (Fig. 34.3). Formal cerebral angiography (Fig. 34.4) showed short focal areas of stenosis in medium-sized arteries. A presumptive diagnosis of vasculitis was made and the patient was treated with steroids. Her headache improved, with further follow-up arranged in her local hospital.

She returned to her home town in another area of the UK, but re-presented with a further thunderclap headache. MRI brain showed no new ischaemic areas but MRA showed focal areas of stenosis that disappeared on follow-up imaging some weeks later.

Questions

1. List the possible causes of thunderclap headache.
2. What is the most likely diagnosis and why?
3. What is the mechanism? Give some causes of this syndrome.
4. What abnormalities may be seen on brain imaging?
5. What is the treatment and prognosis?

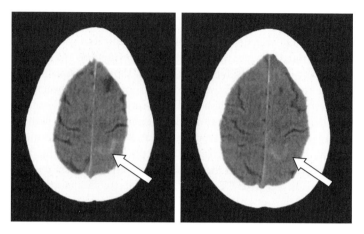

Fig. 34.1 CT brain showing an area of hyperintense material in the cortical sulci at the vertex (arrow). The appearance is consistent with a cortical SAH.

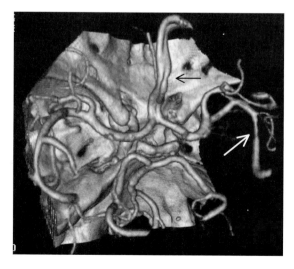

Fig. 34.2 3D CT angiogram showing areas of narrowing in a branch of the left MCA (white arrow) and the left ACA (black arrow).

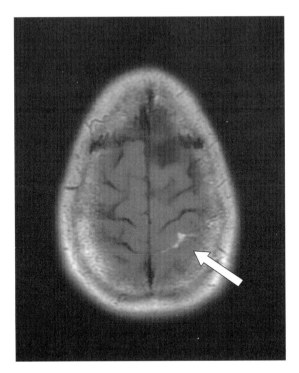

Fig. 34.3 MRI showing area of hyperdense material in the cortical sulci at the vertex previously seen on CT (arrow). The appearance is in keeping with cortical subarachnoid blood.

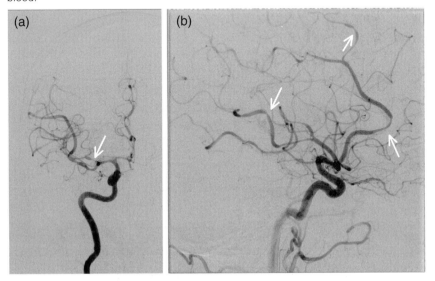

Fig. 34.4 Intra-arterial angiogram: (a) AP view of the right ICA injection and (b) lateral view of the left ICA injection. The arrows indicate narrowing in the right MCA (a), and in the left ACA and MCA (b).

Answers

1. List the possible causes of thunderclap headache.

In any patient presenting with thunderclap headache (i.e. sudden-onset severe headache), SAH must be excluded with a CT scan followed, if negative, by LP performed after 12 hours. If CT and LP are negative, alternative causes should be sought.

The causes of thunderclap headache are listed below.

◆ Vascular
- Haemorrhage
  - aneurysmal SAH
  - peri-mesencephalic SAH
  - other intracranial haemorrhage (especially cerebellar, intraventricular)
- Infarction
  - especially cerebellar
- Cervical artery dissection (see Case 24)
  - especially if pain is lateralized
- Venous sinus thrombosis (see Case 17)
- Giant cell arteritis (see Case 15)
- Reversible cerebral vasoconstriction syndrome
◆ Non-vascular
- Benign thunderclap headache
- Sinusitis
- Meningitis
- Brain tumour
- Low-pressure headache.

2. What is the most likely diagnosis and why?

The most likely diagnosis is reversible cerebral vasoconstriction syndrome (RCVS).

Alternative terms for RCVS include:

◆ Call–Fleming syndrome
◆ benign angiopathy of the CNS
◆ migraine angiitis
◆ idiopathic thunderclap headache with reversible vasospasm
◆ post-partum angiopathy.

This patient went on to have imaging of the cerebral circulation because of concerns over the unusual appearances of the distal carotid arteries.

Table 34.1 Criteria for RCVS

Acute severe headache (often thunderclap) with or without focal neurological deficit or seizures
Monophasic course without new symptoms more than a month after symptom onset
Segmental vasoconstriction on MRA, CTA, or catheter angiography
Resolution of arterial abnormalities within 12 weeks
Exclusion of SAH from ruptured aneurysm
Normal or near-normal CSF

Angiography demonstrated segmental narrowing and dilatation ('string of beads' appearance) of the cerebral vessels. The presence of such angiographic abnormalities which are indistinguishable from cerebral vasculitis, together with a history of thunderclap headache and subsequent resolution of the angiographic changes, is consistent with RCVS (see Table 34.1). Red flags to the diagnosis are shown in Box 34.1.

The headache in RCVS is secondary to the vascular abnormality in contrast with migraine (see Case 7) in which the headache occurs without any causal underlying vascular lesion. A history of migraine is no more common in those with RCVS than in the general population at 16–20%, and those with migraine identify the headache as different from their usual migraine headache. Headache, usually bilateral, is often the only symptom, as illustrated by the case above, and is often, although not invariably, thunderclap in nature. The headache is usually posterior and may be associated with agitation, nausea, photophobia, and phonophobia. Multiple thunderclap headaches occurring on most days over 1–4 weeks are highly suggestive of RCVS, and they may often have a trigger such as sexual activity, coughing, sneezing, or sudden head movement.

Focal deficits and seizures may occur in association with the headache. Deficits may be TIA- or stroke-like in onset or may come on gradually over a few minutes with positive visual or sensory symptoms mimicking migrainous auras. Persistent focal deficits are usually associated with haematoma or infarction (see below). Patients are usually alert, but coma and multiple strokes may occur in severe cases.

3. What is the mechanism? Give some causes of this syndrome.

The mechanism of RCVS is uncertain, but is thought to involve a transient disturbance in the control of cerebral vascular tone leading to focal arterial vasoconstriction and dilatation.

Box 34.1 Red flags to the diagnosis of RCVS

- Multiple thunderclap headache episodes over 1–3 weeks
- Non-aneurysmal SAH, especially if cortical
- Cryptogenic stroke in the presence of severe headache

The disturbance of control of cerebral vascular tone may occur either spontaneously or after exposure to vasoactive substances and/or the post-partum state. Implicated vasoactive substances include selective serotonin reuptake inhibitors, nasal decongestants, some diet pills and herbal remedies, and illicit drugs (cannabis, cocaine, ecstasy, amphetamines). Symptoms may occur after only a few doses or after several months of use. Post-partum RCVS usually starts in the first week after delivery and may be associated with the use of ergot derivatives to treat post-partum haemorrhage or bromocriptine to inhibit lactation. Other causes include catecholamine-secreting tumours (e.g. phaeochromocytoma), and carotid surgery.

Severe forms of RCVS overlap with the posterior reversible encephalopathy syndrome (PRES) in which severe headache is accompanied by confusion, seizures, and cortical blindness, and there is a characteristic imaging pattern on MRI better seen on FLAIR than on T2. There is bilateral symmetrical high signal affecting the cortex, subcortex, and deep white matter, principally of the parieto-occipital regions, but which may also involve the temporo-occipital junction and the posterior fossa and brainstem. This corresponds to areas of reversible vasogenic oedema, although infarction and cytotoxic oedema with restricted diffusion may occur. PRES was first described in association with severe hypertension, often in the setting of eclampsia or ciclosporin therapy, but may also occur in association with transplantation, chemotherapy, or septic shock, or spontaneously. Severe hypertension is thought to result in failure of cerebral autoregulation, although the observation that around 20% of cases are normotensive has led to the proposal that inflammatory mediators may be involved.

4. What abnormalities may be seen on brain imaging?

Brain imaging may show cortical SAH, lobar haemorrhage, or rarely infarction.

In RCVS, non-contrast CT is usually normal, whereas MRI is abnormal in around one-third of cases. Cortical SAH is the most common abnormality, occurring in 20% of cases, and PRES occurs in 10% (cortical SAH may also occur in CAA—see Case 6). In patients with a persistent neurological deficit, haematoma or infarction is seen on MRI. Focal ICH may be single or multiple, cortical or deep, and of variable volume (multiple lobar haemorrhages are also a feature of CAA). Subdural haemorrhage has been reported. Infarction is rare, but may be multiple and often has a border-zone distribution. Symmetrical high signal on FLAIR is consistent with PRES. RCVS should always be considered in the presence of non-aneurysmal SAH (cortical rather than in the typical peri-mesencephalic location) and/or cryptogenic stroke.

Non-invasive angiography (CTA or MRA) is usually sufficient to show the focal restrictions and dilatations of the cerebral vessels. Changes may be seen in both anterior and posterior vessels, may affect large vessels such as the carotid siphon (as seen in this case), and are usually bilateral and widespread. Serial scanning may show a dynamic process with previously narrowed areas normalizing and vice versa. Of note, early angiography (within <5 days of symptom onset) may be normal, and a repeat study may be required some days later.

5. What is the treatment and prognosis?

Treatment is supportive and the prognosis is generally favourable.

Patients require rest for a few days to weeks. A careful history should be taken to identify triggers, including the use of vasoactive substances. Intensive care is required for severe cases. Empirical nimodipine may be given, but there are no randomized data to support its use.

In a typical case, there are multiple attacks of headache within the first week followed by a residual milder headache that disappears within 3 weeks. PRES and intracranial haemorrhage tend to occur within the first week after onset, whereas TIA and ischaemic strokes occur later, often as the headache improves.

The vast majority of patients recover completely, although persistent mild headache and fatigue may continue for some months. Those with stroke may be left with residual disability. Fatalities have been reported, usually in the post-partum setting. The long-term outcome regarding recurrence is uncertain owing to the lack of follow-up studies. The current patient remained well some months later.

Further reading

Ducros A, Bousser M-G (2009). Reversible cerebral vasoconstriction syndrome. *Pract Neurol*; **9**: 256–67.

Case 35

Case 35.A

A 64-year-old female was referred by her GP having reported an episode of visual blurring in her left eye that had occurred one day earlier while she was watching televison. This lasted for only a few seconds but was followed by a sensation that a black curtain was falling over her left eye. This lasted for a few minutes and recovered spontaneously. She had an unremarkable past medical history, was an ex-smoker, and was myopic. Her blood pressure was 150/90mmHg and her pulse was 88bpm and irregular. Fundoscopy revealed grade 1 bilateral hypertensive retinopathy. No murmurs or carotid bruits were heard. An ECG showed AF.

Case 35.B

A 53-year-old woman presented to the TIA clinic with three episodes of right-sided visual loss over the previous 2 weeks. She described this as sudden-onset blackness coming down over her right eye like a curtain. This persisted for 5–10 minutes before her vision returned, although it would remain blurred for another 10–15 minutes. The patient reported that, when she covered her left eye with her hand, she was unable to see anything out of her right eye at all during the episode. When sitting at a computer during an event, she usually turned to the right so that she could make full use of her preserved vision on the left. There were no other symptoms with these attacks, and no subsequent headache. The patient had always been healthy, had kept physically active, and had never smoked. She was not on any medication, and there was no family history of vascular disease.

The patient had carotid Dopplers and a CT brain scan, both of which were reported as normal. She returned for further review 2 months later. At this time she reported that the episodes had persisted, and that she was getting them at least every other day. An MRI brain scan was organized.

Questions

1. What is your differential diagnosis for patient A? And patient B?

2. How would you investigate patient A further and why? How would you manage her further?

3. Patient B's MRI scan is shown in Fig. 35.1. What does it show?

4. What do you now think is the cause of patient B's attacks? How would you manage her further?

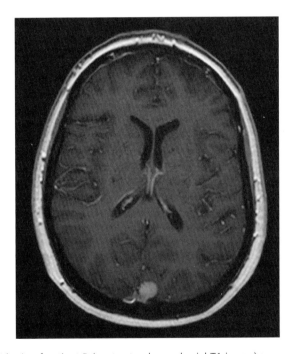

Fig. 35.1 MRI brain of patient B (contrast-enhanced axial T1 image).

Answers

1. What is your differential diagnosis for patient A? And patient B?

Patient A describes one episode of sudden-onset monocular visual loss. The description of 'a curtain coming down' is said to be typical of amaurosis fugax, which is due to transient retinal ischaemia. Such episodes are generally caused by transient embolic occlusion of a retinal artery branch or the central retinal artery. Symptoms usually last for some minutes. The visual disturbance may be fairly non-specific. Patients can describe greying or blackening out of vision, dimming of vision, or sometimes appearances as if looking through broken glass. While a curtain coming down is often described, this is not a definite requirement for the diagnosis. However, symptoms are usually negative, i.e. patients describe a loss of vision rather than additional symptoms such as seeing flashing lights or zigzag lines.

Patient B gives a similar history of one-sided visual loss, which she perceives as monocular. The important differentiating factor is the high number of attacks she experiences. This would be unusual for recurrent ischaemic events, unless they are due to low flow rather than embolism. One might then expect a postural component to the symptoms, in that they would occur mainly in the upright position. Recurrent episodes of monocular visual disturbance may also occur with retinal migraine, although patients often describe positive symptoms, such as zigzag lines or flashing lights. Finally, it is possible that patients perceive visual loss as monocular even though they are experiencing a hemianopia, and they are unable to tell the difference between loss of vision out of one eye and loss of vision in one hemifield. Recurrent episodes of visual disturbance in one hemifield can also be due to transient ischaemia, migraine, or epilepsy. Classically, seizures arising from the visual cortex present with the perception of coloured round shapes. However, ictal blindness has also been described.

2. How would you investigate patient A further and why? How would you manage her further?

Patient A's history is highly suggestive of classical amaurosis fugax due to transient embolic occlusion of the retinal artery. Therefore she should be investigated for embolic sources. The patient's ECG showed AF, and her amaurosis fugax might well have been due to cardioembolism. As AF was a new diagnosis, the patient should have an echocardiogram to look for an underlying structural lesion. More commonly, amaurosis fugax is due to embolism from carotid atheroma. The patient should have carotid imaging, which is usually done with duplex ultrasound. This gives a good view of the carotid bifurcation, which is the most common site of carotid atheroma and is also the most amenable to surgical intervention. Other imaging modalities, such as MRA or CTA, also allow assessment of the more proximal and distal vessel for the presence of any atheromatous plaque and stenosis.

This patient's carotid ultrasound did not show any significant carotid stenosis. Had there been a left ICA stenosis, this would have been the possible cause of her symptoms, and she should have been referred for carotid endarterectomy (see Case 19 for further information on the management of carotid disease). In the absence of carotid atheroma, cardioembolism is the most likely source of her visual disturbance and, if there are no contraindications, she should be anticoagulated to prevent any further cardioembolic events. She should also be referred to cardiology to assess whether she is suitable for cardioversion and for further evaluation of her AF.

3. Patient B's MRI scan is shown in Fig. 35.1. What does it show?

The MRI shows a small well-circumscribed lesion in the left occipital pole. It shows avid regular contrast enhancement. This lesion is a small meningioma.

4. What do you now think is the cause of patient B's attacks? How would you manage her further?

The meningioma is in a location where it may cause visual disturbance in the right visual hemifield. The patient is describing recurrent stereotyped episodes. Even though she is not describing any positive visual phenomena, it is most likely that her symptoms are due to seizures arising from the occipital cortex. It remains unclear why she should have had total loss of vision from her right eye, but her description of turning her chair to the right when looking at a computer screen during an episode may have been an indication that she was describing a hemianopia. Certainly, this case highlights how difficult it can be to differentiate between monocular visual loss and homonymous hemianopia.

As recurrent seizures were now the most likely diagnosis, the patient was started on an anticonvulsant (lamotrigine). Her symptoms settled after she had reached a dose of 75mg twice daily, which was further diagnostic confirmation. The patient was told that, according to DVLA regulations, she must not drive for a year after cessation of symptoms (see also Case 23). The patient should have further follow-up imaging to monitor the meningioma for any increase in size in order to be able to arrange timely further intervention, should this be required, and her visual fields should also be monitored.

Further reading

Panayiotopoulos CP (1999). Visual phenomena and headache in occipital epilepsy: a review, a systematic study and differentiation from migraine. *Epileptic Disord*; 1: 205–16.

Case 36

A 39-year-old woman developed a left ptosis and a pressure feeling behind her left eye over several days. She also became aware of a 'whooshing' sound in her head. Symptoms persisted for 4 weeks. The patient then developed a right-sided headache and neck pain of sudden onset and worsening every day. After 2 weeks, the headache had become unbearable and she was admitted to hospital. On admission, she was alert and orientated. She had a left-sided Horner's syndrome, but no focal neurological deficit. She was afebrile and had no neck stiffness. Blood pressure was 220/110mmHg. The patient's CT angiogram and intra-arterial angiogram are shown in Fig 36.1 and Fig 36.2, respectively.

Questions

1. What do the CT angiogram (Fig. 36.1) and the intra-arterial angiogram (Fig. 36.2) show? How do these findings explain the patient's symptoms?
2. What is the underlying diagnosis?
3. How would you manage this patient acutely?
4. How could this patient's hypertension be related to her imaging findings?
5. How would you manage this patient in the long term?

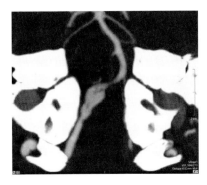

Fig. 36.1 CT angiogram: AP view of the right vertebral artery and the basilar artery.

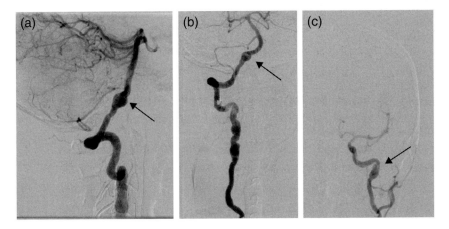

Fig. 36.2 Intra-arterial angiogram, right vertebral artery injection: (a) lateral view and (b) AP view. Panel (c) shows a left ICA injection.

Answers

1. What do the CT angiogram (Fig. 36.1) and the intra-arterial angiogram (Fig. 36.2) show? How do these findings explain the patient's symptoms?

The CTA and intra-arterial angiogram show a dilated right vertebral artery with a string-and-bead appearance and a large pseudo-aneurysm in the distal vessel close to the vertebrobasilar junction. The intra-arterial angiogram also shows a dissection of the left ICA at the C1/C2 level. The left ICA dissection is the most likely explanation for the patient's Horner's syndrome. The associated vessel stenosis causes turbulent blood flow, which explains the patient's perception of a pulse-synchronous 'whooshing' sound. The patient's headache is most likely explained by the vertebral artery dissection and development of a pseudo-aneurysm. The worsening of the headache indicates that the aneurysm is expanding and that the vessel walls are being increasingly stretched. Rupture of the aneurysm may be imminent. This is a life-threatening situation.

2. What is the underlying diagnosis?

The underlying diagnosis is FMD (see Case 5). This is a non-inflammatory non-atheromatous vasculopathy affecting small and medium-sized arteries. It can affect all layers of the vessel wall, though it most frequently affects the media. The structure of the media becomes disorganized. There are alternating areas of thinning of the media and thickened fibromuscular ridges, which lead to the string-and-bead appearance of the vessel. The disease most commonly affects young and middle-aged women. It can occur in every arterial bed, but most frequently affects the renal and cerebral vessels where it can cause stenosis, spontaneous dissections, and aneurysms. The aetiology of the disease is uncertain. Some authors have suggested that it may be an inherited disorder with an autosomal dominant inheritance pattern, but others have only rarely found a familial association. It is possible that it is a common presentation of heterogeneous disorders. Certainly, the appearance of FMD has been described in association with other disorders, for example Marfan's syndrome, Ehlers–Danlos syndrome type IV, α_1-antitrypsin deficiency, phaeochromocytoma, and Takayasu's arteritis. Therefore if a patient presents with features of FMD, these conditions should always be considered.

3. How would you manage this patient acutely?

First and foremost this patient's aneurysm needed to be treated. The increasing pain indicated that the aneurysm was expanding and might have been about to rupture. Therefore treatment had to commence as soon as possible. Treatment options included occlusion of the vertebral artery, or coiling and stenting of the aneurysm. Occlusion of the artery would have been the most definitive treatment, but it would only have been possible if the patient had sufficient collateral circulation, as otherwise the occlusion might have caused a brainstem stroke. Our patient had a dominant right vertebral artery and only a very small left vertebral artery with hardly any cross-flow from the anterior circulation via the posterior communicating arteries. Therefore it was extremely unlikely that she would have tolerated the occlusion of her dominant right vertebral artery. Normally, if an arterial occlusion is considered, the patient would first undergo a temporary balloon occlusion of the artery to assess whether there is sufficient functional collateral blood flow, and whether she could tolerate the occlusion without any deficit. However, in this patient the collateral flow was so poor that the test occlusion was not even attempted. Instead, the patient underwent stenting of the aneurysm. This preserved the vessel, but diverted blood flow away from the aneurysm wall. Coils were inserted between the vessel wall and the stent to enhance thrombus formation and scarring and thus prevent further aneurysm formation(Fig. 36.3). The patient tolerated the procedure well and did not develop any complications.

The patient was extremely hypertensive on admission, and this hypertension persisted. High blood pressure increases the risk of aneurysm rupture, and therefore her blood pressure needed to be lowered urgently. This was achieved with a Ca antagonist (amlodipine). A β-blocker (labetalol, which can be given intravenously) would also have been possible, but was relatively contraindicated as a phaeochromocytoma had not yet been excluded, and β-blockade in a phaeochromocytoma may lead to unopposed α-agonism and extreme refractory hypertension. After treatment

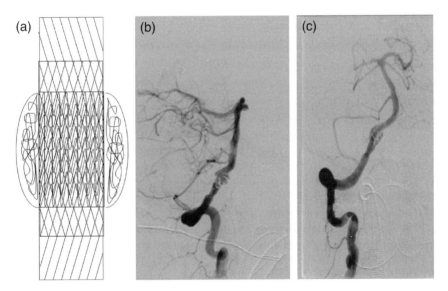

Fig. 36.3 (a) The arrangement of stents and coils used to treat the patient's aneurysm. A stent is deployed distally and proximally to the aneurysm. Coils are inserted into the aneurysm to promote thrombus formation. A further stent is deployed in the aneurysm, overlapping with the two other stents. This ensures vessel patency and blood flow. The aneurysm wall is now isolated from the blood flow, which should prevent further aneurysm growth and rupture. Panels (b) and (c) show the final result of the procedure on the angiogram.

of the aneurysm, the patient had to be investigated for the cause of her hypertension. A further management issue was her ICA dissection. As discussed in Case 24, it is not clear if cervical artery dissections are best treated with anticoagulation or with antiplatelet agents. This patient had not had a cerebral ischaemic event, and the dissection had probably occurred 6 weeks earlier when she developed the Horner's syndrome. It was likely that there had already been some spontaneous healing. Furthermore, the patient was going to be on dual antiplatelet therapy for at least 3 months following her stent insertion. This would also reduce any remaining risk of embolization from her carotid dissection.

4. How could this patient's hypertension be related to her imaging findings?

FMD commonly affects the renal arteries and can cause renal artery stenosis, which in turn can cause hypertension. This patient underwent imaging of her renal arteries, and a left renal artery stenosis was found and treated with angioplasty. Her blood pressure improved very rapidly, though it remained slightly elevated. Another possible explanation for an association of the imaging findings with this patient's hypertension could have been the presence of a phaeochromocytoma, which has been associated with the appearance of FMD as well as the presence of poorly controlled hypertension. However, we found no evidence of a phaeochromocytoma in this patient.

5. How would you manage this patient in the long term?

This patient is at risk of developing further aneurysms and arterial dissections, and of having cerebral ischaemic events due to vascular stenosis or embolization from thrombosed aneurysms or dissections. She may also develop further renal artery stenosis and her hypertension may recur. Follow-up data from patients with FMD are rare, and it is difficult to put a number to these risks. However, it appears that the risk of ischaemic events is lower than in patients with stenosis due to atheromatous disease. Nevertheless, as the patient also has her vertebral stents, she should remain on lifelong antiplatelet therapy. Her blood pressure should be monitored closely. If she re-develops hypertension, her renal arteries should be imaged again. There are no reliable data on the risk of developing further dissections or aneurysms. The threshold for re-imaging the craniocervical vessels if the patient develops appropriate symptoms should be low. Initially, the patient will undergo repeat imaging to ensure that her vertebral artery aneurysm does not recur. This can also be used to monitor the occurrence of any other new abnormalities. If none occur, the intervals between imaging reviews will increase, but some authors have recommended six-monthly long-term imaging follow-up to monitor any disease progression.

Further reading

Olin JW, Pierce M (2008). Contemporary management of fibromuscular dysplasia. *Curr Opin Cardiol*; **23**: 527–36.

Plouin PF, Perdu J, La Batide-Alanore A, *et al.* (2007). Fibromuscular dysplasia. *Orphanet J Rare Dis*; **2**: 28–35.

Case 37

A 90-year-old man was referred by his GP to the emergency TIA clinic with sudden-onset right arm weakness 2 days previously, accompanied by discomfort over the top of his head. He had subsequently had difficulty shaving and performing fine motor tasks with his right arm. He had otherwise been feeling well. He had a past history of hypertension but no other risk factors for cerebrovascular disease. He was taking aspirin (started by the GP on the day after symptom onset), bendroflumethiazide, and candesartan.

On examination he was well and fit for his age. The head discomfort had resolved. Pulse was 50bpm regular and blood pressure was 140/80mmHg. There was an ejection systolic murmur audible throughout the praecordium, but heart sounds were otherwise normal. There was very mild pyramidal distribution weakness of the right upper limb but no other neurological abnormality.

Investigations showed the following:

◆ Hb 12.0; WCC 5.49; platelets 216; ESR 88; CRP 28; LFTs, Ca, thyroid function normal

◆ Carotid Dopplers: no significant stenosis

◆ ECG: sinus rhythm, left ventricular hypertrophy

◆ MRI brain: see Fig. 37.1. CE-MRA of the cervical and proximal intracranial vessels did not show any significant stenosis.

Questions—Part 1

1. What does the MRI scan show?
2. What are the most likely causes of this patient's stroke?

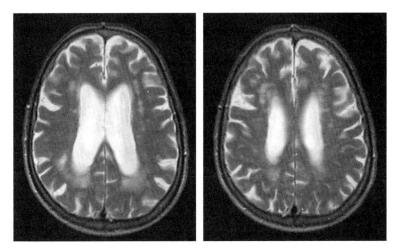

Fig. 37.1 T2-weighted MRI brain.

Answers

1. What does the MRI scan show?

The MRI brain shows widespread periventricular and deep white matter hyperintensities (see Fig. 37.2 with arrows) in keeping with small vessel disease (see Cases 6 and 9).

2. What are the most likely causes of this patient's stroke?

The most likely causes of this patient's cerebral ischaemia are:

◆ small vessel disease

◆ cardioembolism (see Table 37.1).

The absence of significant stenosis on the carotid Doppler and the normal MRA makes large vessel atherothromboembolism unlikely. GCA (see Case 15) causes a large vessel vasculitis in older people and may cause stroke, most commonly in the posterior circulation distribution. GCA was considered in this man owing to the raised inflammatory markers, but he had normal temporal arteries to palpation and his head discomfort was mild and only present at the time of stroke onset, having resolved by the time he presented to the clinic. Furthermore, he had no constitutional symptoms. The MRI scan shows changes consistent with small vessel disease which, together with the history of hypertension, suggest the possibility of stroke secondary to small vessel disease (see Case 49).

The presence of an ejection systolic murmur together with left ventricular hypertrophy raises the possibility of aortic stenosis, although the pulse pressure and heart sounds were normal, making severe stenotic disease less likely. However, the presence of a raised ESR and CRP together with a murmur means that infective endocarditis (IE) should be excluded. Endocarditis can be relatively asymptomatic and may present with stroke (see Case 47). Finally, occult AF may have occurred. Increasing age and hypertension are both strongly associated with AF (see Case 22), and they are both present in this patient.

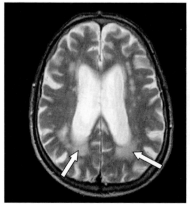 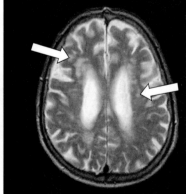

Fig. 37.2 T2-weighted MRI brain showing widespread periventricular (small arrows) and deep white matter hyperintensities (large arrows) in keeping with small vessel disease.

Table 37.1 Causes of cardioembolism

Left atrium

    Atrial fibrillation

    Sinoatrial disease

    Myxoma

    Inter-atrial septal aneurysm

Mitral valve

    Infective endocarditis

    Non-bacterial thrombotic (marantic) endocarditis

    Rheumatic disease

    Prosthetic valve

    Mitral annulus calcification

    Libman–Sacks endocarditis

    Papillary fibroelastoma

Aortic valve

    Infective endocarditis

    Non-bacterial thrombotic or marantic endocarditis

    Rheumatic disease

    Prosthetic valve

    Calcification and/or sclerosis

    Syphilis

Left ventricular mural thrombus

    Myocardial infarction

    Left ventricular aneurysm

    Cardiomyopathy

    Myxoma

    Blunt chest injury

    Mechanical artificial heart

Paradoxical embolism from the venous system

    Atrial septal defect

    Ventricular septal defect

    Patent foramen ovale

    Pulmonary arteriovenous fistula

(continued)

Table 37.1 (continued) Causes of cardioembolism

Congenital cardiac disorders, particularly with right to left shunt
Cardiac surgery
Catheterization
Angioplasty
Others
Primary oxalosis
Hydatid cyst

Questions—Part 2

3. This man went on to have an echocardiogram (Fig. 37.3). What is indicated by the arrow on the echocardiogram?
4. What further investigations are indicated?

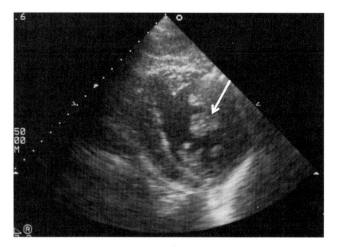

Fig. 37.3 Transthoracic echocardiogram.

Answers

3. This man went on to have an echocardiogram (Fig. 37.3). What is indicated by the arrow on the echocardiogram?

The echocardiogram shows a mass within the left ventricle. The raised ESR suggested a cardiac myxoma, but the lack of constitutional symptoms was not consistent with this diagnosis.

4. What further investigations are indicated?

Further cardiac investigations are required to investigate the cardiac mass.

Cardiac tumours present with symptoms including those related to obstruction, embolism, and constitutional symptoms. Myxomas, especially those with an irregular surface, and papillary fibroelastomas have a high rate of embolism. Cardiac masses can be evaluated using transoesophageal echocardiography or cardiac MRI. Transoesophageal echocardiography has the best spatial and temporal resolution of the cardiac imaging modalities, providing excellent anatomical and functional information, but it is an interventional procedure which requires sedation. This man underwent cardiac MRI which confirmed a cardiac mass arising from the papillae of the left ventricle consistent with a fibroelastoma. Repeat ESR was 22mm/h and CRP was <2mg/L, and it transpired that he had developed an episode of gout soon after his first clinic visit. The cardiologists felt that the fibroelastoma had probably been present for a number of years.

Cardiac tumours are rare. Myxomas are the most common tumour type, followed by sarcoma and fibroelastoma. Echocardiography is currently the preferred diagnostic modality, and MRI and CT are helpful in the differential diagnosis of cardiac tumours. Papillary fibroelastomas can become quite large, and can occur on any valve surface or area of the endocardium. There is no gender predominance and there is a wide range of ages at presentation, with a mean age of approximately 60 years. Fibroelastomas are usually detected incidentally on echocardiography, but left-sided lesions may present with embolic phenomena, resulting in stroke and myocardial infarction. Most symptoms arise from left-sided lesions that shower fibrin clots into the cerebral circulation or prolapse into the coronary orifice. Surgical treatment is advocated by some, especially if embolism has occurred or the tumour is mobile, as tumour mobility is thought to increase the risk of death or embolization.

Cardiac myxomas may be familial and arise in any heart chamber, but 75% are found in the left atrium. Tumour material, or complicating thrombus, may embolize and there are often features of intracardiac obstruction (dyspnoea, cardiac failure, syncope) and constitutional upset (malaise, weight loss, fever, rash, arthralgia, myalgia, anaemia, raised ESR, hyper-gammaglobulinaemia). Myxomatous emboli impacted in cerebral arteries may cause aneurysmal dilatation with subsequent ICH or SAH. Because embolization is the major complication of a myxoma, especially of myxoid friable familial ones, identification of first-degree relatives of patients with documented myxoma syndrome is important.

There is little evidence to guide secondary prevention in stroke associated with cardiac abnormalities other than AF, although atrial myxomas will usually need to be resected. This patient was prescribed aspirin and a statin and his hypertension treatment was closely monitored. It remained unclear (as is frequently the case in stroke where there is more than one possible cause) whether his stroke was caused by small vessel disease or cardioembolism. Given his advanced age, and the uncertain association between the fibroelastoma and the stroke, surgical removal of the tumour was not felt to be appropriate. The patient had no recurrent events over the following year.

Further reading

Burke A, Jeudy J Jr, Virmani R (2008). Cardiac tumours: an update: Cardiac tumours. *Heart*; **94**: 117–23.

Ekinci EI, Donnan GA (2004). Neurological manifestations of cardiac myxoma: a review of the literature and report of cases. *Intern Med J*; **34**: 243–9.

Gowda RM, Khan IA, Nair CK, Mehta NJ, Vasavada BC, Sacchi TJ (2003). Cardiac papillary fibroelastoma: a comprehensive analysis of 725 cases. *Am Heart J*; **146**: 404–10.

Sastre-Garriga J, Molina C, Montaner J, *et al.* (2000). Mitral papillary fibroelastoma as a cause of cardiogenic embolic stroke: report of two cases and review of the literature. *Eur J Neurol*; **7**: 449–53.

Wolf RC, Spiess J, Vasic N, Huber R (2007). Valvular strands and ischemic stroke. *Eur Neurol*; **57**: 227–31.

Case 38

A 61-year-old woman developed attacks of rhythmic arm shaking. Her attacks consisted of briefly feeling dizzy after which her left arm began to shake at a rate of about 3Hz. This lasted from a few seconds up to 2 minutes. Consciousness was never impaired and there were no other symptoms. The attacks were often provoked by standing up and could be terminated by lying down. On average, they occurred once a week. The patient had a history of diabetes, ischaemic heart disease, hypertension, and peripheral vascular disease. She had also had a cardiac pacemaker inserted for second-degree heart block a few months prior to the onset of her attacks. There was no focal neurological deficit, but fundoscopy showed asymmetrical ischaemic retinopathy.

Investigations showed the following:

- CT brain: some atrophy and white matter disease; no focal lesion
- Inter-ictal EEG: normal
- Carotid Doppler: occlusion of the right ICA; 60% stenosis of the left ICA
- 48-hour ECG: no significant pauses or arrhythmias.

Questions

1. What is the diagnosis?
2. Which main alternative diagnosis would you consider? Describe the differentiating features between these two conditions.
3. Which treatment options are available? What is the aim of treatment?

Answers

1. What is the diagnosis?

This woman had low-flow TIAs, also often referred to as 'limb-shaking TIAs'. This is an unusual form of TIA which occurs in patients with severe carotid occlusive disease. They are often brought on by postural change, and can sometimes be relieved by sitting or lying down. Despite this postural relationship, there is usually no associated postural drop in blood pressure. The exact mechanism of the limb movements is unclear, but their association with severe carotid disease and postural change, and the fact that they often improve after revascularization procedures, suggests that they are due to transient focal haemodynamic failure. Cerebral blood flow and vasomotor reactivity are often reduced distal to the occluded artery. Why this should produce limb shaking is uncertain. In syncope, bilateral clonic jerks can occur and are thought to be due to subcortical release phenomena caused by diffuse cortical hypoxia. It has been suggested that the limb movements in low-flow TIAs are a focal manifestation of the same process.

2. Which main alternative diagnosis would you consider? Describe the differentiating features between these two conditions.

The main differential diagnosis, which was also considered in this patient, are focal motor seizures (see Case 23). Clinically, the main differentiating features are that there is no Jacksonian march in limb-shaking TIAs, and that they do not extend to the face. They are often associated with postural change, whereas focal motor seizures are not. EEG recordings during limb-shaking TIAs do not show epileptic discharges and, if a treatment trial is done, anticonvulsants are usually ineffective.

3. Which treatment options are available? What is the aim of treatment?

As low-flow TIAs are associated with carotid occlusive disease, they carry a high risk of stroke. The aim of treatment is twofold: to reduce the risk of stroke and to abolish the symptoms, both of which can be achieved by maintaining or improving cerebral blood flow. Management focuses on careful control of blood pressure and on surgical revascularization. In several cases an improvement of symptoms has been reported after raising blood pressure. However, this may be harmful in the presence of concomitant cardiac and renal disease. In such cases, more aggressive treatment of hypertension is possible after surgical revascularization, which is also effective in abolishing the attacks. In patients with an internal carotid stenosis, endarterectomy is the procedure of choice to abolish symptoms and reduce stroke risk. In patients with complete occlusion, extracranial–intracranial bypass surgery may stop the attacks, although there is no evidence that it reduces the risk of stroke.

Further reading

Niehaus L, Neuhauser H, Meyer BU (1998). TIAs of hemodynamic origin mimicking simple partial motor seizures. *Nervenarzt*; **69**: 901–4.

Schulz UG, Rothwell PM (2002). Transient ischaemic attacks mimicking focal motor seizures. *Postgrad Med J*; **78**: 246–7.

Tatemichi TK, Young WL, Prohovnik I, *et al.* Perfusion insufficiency in limb-shaking transient ischemic attacks. *Stroke*; 1990; **21**: 341.

Case 39

An 83-year-old woman was admitted to the physicians from the acute psychiatric ward for the elderly where she had been admitted with confusion on a background of anxiety and depression. There was a past history of an oesophageal web. Medications were olanzapine, venlafaxine, trazodone, simvastatin, Fybogel, senna, and lorazepam. On examination, she was apyrexial, pulse 70bpm, and blood pressure 120/70mmHg. She was mildly confused (MMSE 20/30) and complaining of headache. Neurological examination revealed a right homonymous hemianopia.

Investigations showed the following:

◆ Na 126; CRP 60

◆ CT brain: reported as showing an acute occipito-parietal infarct

◆ TTE: aortic sclerosis, no evidence of mass or vegetation

The patient was started on aspirin and simvastatin for secondary prevention after a presumed stroke. The following day she was noted to be flushed with a temperature of 37.6°C, although she remained otherwise cardiovascularly stable, and blood and urine cultures were requested. She was started on oral antibiotics for a presumed chest infection. Over the next 2 days, she became increasingly confused and non-compliant with examination. Her GCS dropped to 13–14/15. The CT brain scans were re-reviewed by a neuroradiologist, and CT with contrast was requested (see Fig. 39.1).

Questions

1. Why might the patient have become confused?

2. What does the CT with contrast show? What is the differential diagnosis based on the scan findings (Fig. 39.1)?

3. What would you do next?

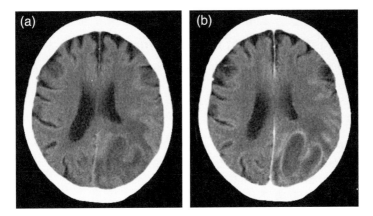

Fig. 39.1 CT brain scan without contrast (a) and after contrast administration (b).

Answers

1. Why might the patient have become confused?

The possible causes of confusion in this patient are:

- systemic infection and delirium
- delirium secondary to stroke (see Case 43)
- CNS infection
- hyponatraemia.

Delirium (acute confusional state characterized by altered level of consciousness, inattention, fluctuation and disordered thinking) is common in frail elderly patients. The aetiology is usually multifactorial, and delirium is most common in those with prior cognitive impairment. There was no definite previous history of cognitive impairment in this patient, but she had been admitted with anxiety and depression which are more common in those with impaired cognition. Stroke is also associated with delirium (see Case 43) and could have been the cause in this case. However, this patient's continuing decline in level of consciousness, together with raised inflammatory markers and pyrexia, should make one question whether stroke alone could be responsible. In this case, the original brain imaging was reviewed, and in retrospect the original diagnosis of stroke was wrong.

2. What does the CT with contrast show? What is the differential diagnosis based on the scan findings?

The CT with contrast shows an enhancing lesion in the left occipitoparietal lesion consistent with a tumour (glioblastoma multiforme) or an abscess (Fig. 39.2).

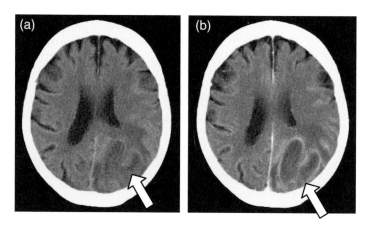

Fig. 39.2 CT brain scan showing an enhancing lesion in the left parieto-occipital region consistent with a tumour (glioblastoma multiforme) or an abscess.

3. What would you do next?

The patient needs an urgent neurosurgical referral. Aspirin and simvastatin should be stopped. Intravenous ceftriaxone and metronidazole should be started. Further neuroimaging should be performed (MRI).

MRI showed a space-occupying lesion with high signal on DWI, indicative of cytotoxic oedema. This showed that the lesion was an abscess rather than a tumour with vasogenic oedema, which would not have high signal on DWI (Fig. 39.3). The abscess was aspirated and Gram stain showed Gram-positive cocci. Subsequent culture confirmed *Streptococcus milleri*. It was hypothesized that the patient might have aspirated as a result of her oesophageal web and developed a lower respiratory tract infection which was the source of the cerebral abscess. Subsequent repeat CT over the next 2 months showed reduction and then resolution of the abscess (Fig. 39.4).

This case illustrates the importance of revisiting the diagnosis when the patient's condition changes or when the clinical features do not fit (see also Cases 1 and 30). In particular, cerebral imaging should always be reviewed with an experienced radiologist if there is any doubt about the diagnosis.

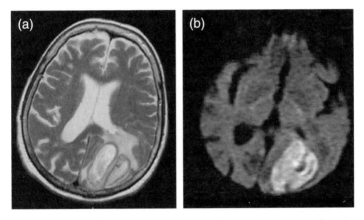

Fig. 39.3 MRI brain. (a) The T2-weighted image shows a left-sided parieto-occipital space-occupying lesion with peri-lesional oedema and compression of the left lateral ventricle. Appearances would be in keeping with a high-grade tumour, such as a glioblastoma, or with a cerebral abscess. (b) DWI shows high signal within the lesion, consistent with cytotoxic oedema. These appearances indicate that the lesion is an abscess rather than a tumour.

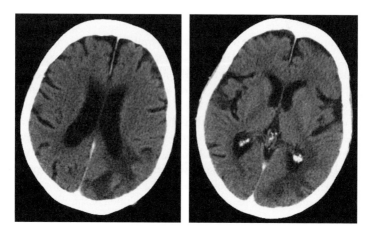

Fig. 39.4 CT brain after 2 weeks of intravenous antibiotics, showing partial resolution of the abscess.

Further reading

Foerster BR, Thurnher MM, Malani PN, Petrou M, Carets-Zumelzu F, Sundgren PC (2007). Intracranial infections: clinical and imaging characteristics. *Acta Radiol*; **48**: 875–93.

Romano A, Bozzao A, Bonamini M, *et al.* (2003). Diffusion-weighted MR imaging: clinical applications in neuroradiology. *Radiol Med*; **106**: 521–48.

Shintani S, Tsuruoka S, Koumo Y, Shiigai T (1996). Sudden 'stroke-like' onset of homonymous hemianopsia due to bacterial brain abscess. *J Neurol Sci*; **143**: 190–4.

Wispelwey B, Scheld WM (1992). Brain abscess. *Semin Neurol*; **12**: 273–8.

Case 40

A 22-year-old man presented to the neurology clinic with poorly controlled epilepsy. The patient had been diagnosed with epilepsy at the age of 6 years. At this time, a CT brain scan had shown right frontal scarring, presumed to be due to perinatal ischaemia. He may have had generalized tonic–clonic seizures, but only very few details were available. He used to have approximately one seizure per year. More recently the patient described a change in his attacks. They consisted of his left hand shaking, sometimes associated with a feeling of his head moving up and down, light-headedness, and fatigue. An eyewitness also described occasional associated agitated behaviour. It was unclear if there was any loss of consciousness, although after an attack the patient often 'went to sleep' for 30 minutes. The frequency of these attacks had recently increased to one a month. Several anticonvulsants were tried, but the attack frequency remained unchanged.

Over the next few months, the patient developed attacks of unilateral throbbing headache. These occurred almost daily, lasted 2–3 hours, and were at times associated with scintillating scotomata affecting both eyes. The headache did not respond to treatment with triptan drugs or non-steroidal anti-inflammatory drugs. The patient eventually attended for an MRI brain scan (Fig. 40.1) and a subsequent intra-arterial angiogram (Fig. 40.2).

Questions

1. What is your differential diagnosis for the attacks experienced by this patient?
2. Describe the abnormalities on the MRI brain scan and the intra-arterial angiogram.
3. What is the diagnosis?
4. At what age does this condition usually present? Describe the typical presenting features.
5. Describe the prognosis and available treatment options.

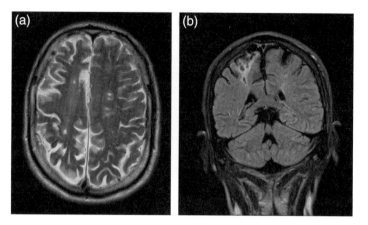

Fig. 40.1 MRI brain. Axial T2-weighted image (a) and the coronal FLAIR image (b).

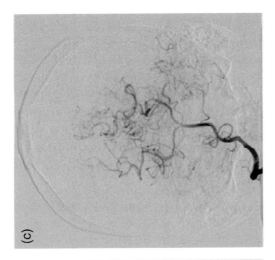

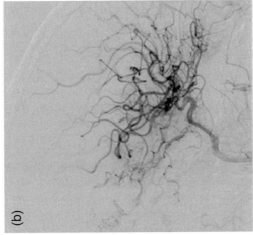

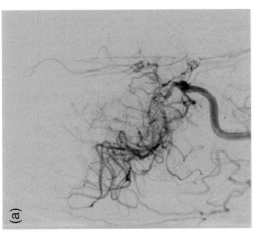

Fig. 40.2 Intra-arterial angiogram: (a) AP view and (b) lateral view of a right ICA injection. (c) A right vertebral artery injection.

Answers

1. What is your differential diagnosis for the attacks experienced by this patient?

The main differential diagnosis is between focal onset seizures (case 23) and low-flow phenomena. The patient has a right frontal cortical scar, which may be the underlying lesion for focal seizures, and which may previously have caused secondary generalized seizures. The confusion and, in particular, the patient going to sleep after an attack would also be in keeping with epilepsy. However, it is possible that the patient's attacks represent low-flow TIAs. These can occur in severe vascular occlusive disease and may present with limb shaking (see also Cases 15 and 38) The apparent confusion may represent dysphasia—it is often difficult to tell the difference between confusion and dysphasia when taking the history. However, going to sleep after an attack is not usually a feature of transient ischaemia. The most helpful investigation in diagnosing the nature of the attacks would be to get an EEG during an attack, preferably with video recording, as this should show epileptic discharges if the attacks were epileptic in nature. An EEG when the patient is symptom free is less likely to be helpful, and it may well also show abnormalities over the cortical scar and those due to chronic underlying hypoperfusion. The other way to find out if the attacks are epileptic would be to start treating the patient with anticonvulsants and monitor his response. TIAs should not improve with anticonvulsants.

2. Describe the abnormalities on the MRI brain scan and the intra-arterial angiogram.

The MRI shows cerebral atrophy and multiple small infarcts in the corona radiata. Both the axial T2-weighted image (Fig. 40.1(a)) and the coronal FLAIR image (Fig. 40.1(b)) show a chronic infarct in the watershed territory of the right middle and anterior cerebral arteries with some haemorrhagic transformation. The intra-arterial angiogram (Fig 40.2) shows high-grade stenoses of the anterior and middle cerebral arteries, distended small lenticulostriate arteries, and numerous other collaterals ((a) and (b)). The right vertebral artery injection (c) shows extensive filling of leptomeningeal collaterals. The appearance of stenosis of the large vessels in the anterior circulation, distended lenticulostriate arteries, and leptomeningeal collaterals is typical of moyamoya disease.

3. What is the diagnosis?

The diagnosis is moyamoya disease. This is a rare condition that was initially thought to affect mainly people of Japanese heritage. However, over recent years it has also been described in populations of other ethnic backgrounds. The main feature of moyamoya disease is progressive stenosis of the terminal internal carotid arteries and the proximal anterior and middle cerebral arteries. The reduced flow through these vessels leads to the formation of small collateral vessels predominantly via branches of the external carotid arteries. On angiography, these vessels give the appearance of a 'puff of smoke', which in Japanese is 'moyamoya'. In moyamoya disease, the carotid arteries gradually occlude for no obvious reason. There is also 'moyamoya syndrome', in which there is a similar radiological appearance, but there are other causative factors associated with the vasculopathy, for example atheroma, previous radiotherapy, or vasculitis.

The diagnosis of moyamoya syndrome is made with vascular imaging, which typically shows bilateral stenosis or occlusion of the distal internal carotid arteries and the proximal anterior and middle cerebral arteries. Intra-arterial angiography is still the gold standard, but MRA and CTA are also helpful. There are a number of conditions which are associated with moyamoya syndrome such as prior radiotherapy to the head, Down's syndrome, sickle cell disease, and neurofibromatosis type 1, and also atheroma or vasculitis. Many of these conditions have already been diagnosed when a diagnosis of moyamoya is made. However, if the condition causing the moyamoya syndrome is thought to be atheroma or vasculitis, this should be investigated further and treated accordingly. Further investigations may also be directed at assessing vascular reserve and cerebral perfusion. This may be useful in predicting which patients may benefit from surgical intervention, and in assessing the effect of surgery by measuring perfusion before and after the intervention. However, it is not clear if such investigations really do provide prognostic information.

4. At what age does this condition usually present? Describe the typical presenting features.

There are two age peaks at which moyamoya disease presents. The first peak is in childhood, between 5 and 9 years. The second peak is in adulthood in patients aged about 40 years. The clinical presentation differs between these patient groups: whereas children frequently present with ischaemic symptoms, about half of adult patients experience cerebral haemorrhage. The presentation with both ischaemic and haemorrhagic events is characteristic of moyamoya disease and should make one consider this condition. Generally the presenting features in moyamoya disease can be attributed to complications of vascular occlusion (TIA, ischaemic stroke, post-stroke epilepsy) and complications of neovascularization and collateralization (haemorrhage arising from fragile new vessels, headache from dilated meningeal vessels). Some patients, particularly children, may develop cognitive and behavioural problems, most likely due to persistent frontal lobe ischaemia or infarction. Abnormal movements, again more commonly occurring in children, are another presenting feature.

5. Describe the prognosis and available treatment options.

Generally, moyamoya disease will progress if left untreated, although the rate of progression may vary considerably between patients. The disease may progress very slowly, with rare subsequent events, or it can have a fulminant course with rapid decline. There is no effective medical treatment for moyamoya disease. Many centres use aspirin to prevent emboli from small thrombi that form at the site of the vascular stenoses, although this could be a potential problem in patients with cerebral haemorrhage. Any medication that lowers blood pressure should only be used cautiously to avoid cerebral hypoperfusion. Regardless of any medical treatment, about two-thirds of patients with conservative treatment will have symptomatic progression over 5 years,. In contrast, only 2–3% of patients who undergo surgical treatment are reported to experience progression.

There are two main ways of treating moyamoya disease surgically: direct and indirect revascularization. In direct revascularization, a branch of the external carotid artery is anastomosed with a cortical branch of the middle or anterior cerebral artery. In indirect revascularization procedures, vascular tissue that is supplied by the external carotid artery (e.g. superficial temporalis muscle) is placed directly onto the cerebral cortex. Over some weeks, this leads to growth of new blood vessels into the underlying cortex. Generally, direct revascularization is done in adult patients who would benefit from rapid reinstitution of blood flow. An indirect approach is usually preferred in children, who have smaller blood vessels that are more difficult to anastomose. In some centres, direct and indirect approaches are combined.

Further reading

Kuroda S, Houkin K (2008). Moyamoya disease: current concepts and future perspectives. *Lancet Neurol*; 7: 1056–66.

Scott RM, Smith ER (2009). Moyamoya disease and moyamoya syndrome. *N Eng J Med*; 360: 1226–37.

Case 41

A 69-year-old retired businesswoman was referred to the emergency TIA clinic on return from a holiday in Switzerland. Four days before returning to the UK, she had developed sudden onset of right facial droop, slurred speech, and difficulty in expressing herself although she was able to understand her husband. The speech difficulty lasted for 24 hours but the dysarthria and facial weakness persisted. There was a past history of Crohn's disease and this had flared up a couple of days prior to developing the neurological deficit. She also mentioned infrequent palpitations over the preceding 6 months. Additional past history included hypertension and renal impairment. She did not seek medical review in Switzerland, but took some additional Pentasa medication. Her medications were clopidogrel 75mg/day, folic acid 5mg/day, ramipril 5mg/day, and Pentasa MR 1000mg twice daily.

On examination, pulse was 77bpm (regular), blood pressure was 170/75mmHg, and heart sounds were normal. There was a mild right facial upper motor neuron weakness and dysarthria.

Investigations showed the following:

◆ Blood tests: Hb 10.9; ESR 39; CRP 3; total cholesterol 5.4; triglycerides 1.29

◆ ECG: sinus rhythm with partial right bundle branch block

◆ Carotid Doppler: left ICA <40% stenosis; right ICA 40–45% stenosis

◆ Echocardiogram: dilated left atrium, otherwise unremarkable; normal left ventricular systolic function; normal right heart

◆ CT brain (Fig. 41.1)

◆ MRI brain (Fig. 41.2)

◆ MRA cervical vessels (Fig. 41.3)

◆ Five-day ECG monitoring (Reveal® test): sinus rhythm with frequent episodes of PAF.

Questions

1. What are the possible causes of this patient's cerebrovascular event?
2. What is the significance of the microbleeds?
3. Would you warfarinize this patient?

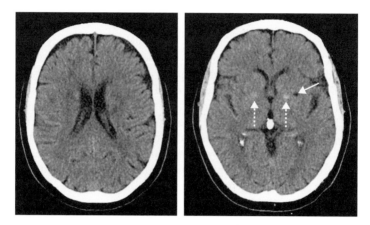

Fig. 41.1 CT brain shows a left-sided lacunar infarct in the lentiform nucleus (solid arrow). There is mild small vessel disease and some calcification of the basal ganglia (dashed arrows).

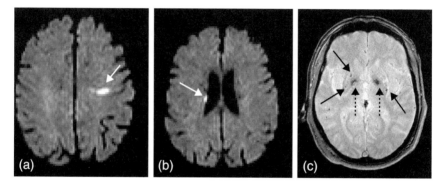

Fig. 41.2 Acute infarct in the subcortical white matter of the left frontal lobe (a) related to the precentral gyrus in keeping with a MCA perforator artery territory infarct, further small acute MCA perforator artery territory infarct adjacent to the right lateral ventricle in the deep white matter (b). GRE (c) also shows multiple microhaemorrhages bilaterally (solid arrows) and the basal ganglia calcification (dashed arrows).

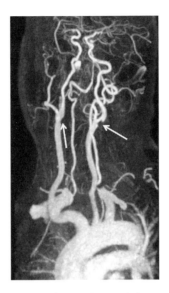

Fig. 41.3 MRA shows bilateral internal carotid stenosis (arrows). The vertebrobasilar system is normal.

Answers

1. What are the possible causes of this patient's cerebrovascular event?

The most likely cause of her strokes is small vessel disease.

The brain imaging shows lateral MCA perforator territory infarcts with moderate bilateral ICA origin stenoses. The infarcts are most likely microvascular, but given that there are two acute infarcts in different territories and evidence of PAF, a cardiac cause cannot be excluded. However, it is rare for cardioembolism to cause subcortical infarctions. Likewise, large vessel disease and thromboembolism are possible, but the territory of infarction suggests that small vessel disease is a more likely cause.

2. What is the significance of the microbleeds?

Brain microbleeds (BMBs) are small homogeneous round foci of low signal intensity on haem-sensitive gradient echo (GRE or T2*) sequences on MRI which represent perivascular collections of haemosiderin deposits. Using conventional MR sequences, the prevalence of BMBs is about 5% in healthy people but increases with age. Microbleeds are associated with stroke: overall around 34% of patients with ischaemic strokes and 60% with haemorrhagic strokes have microbleeds. The prevalence is less in first ever compared with recurrent strokes, suggesting that BMBs are a marker for severity of the underlying cerebrovascular disease. Microbleeds are particularly common in CAA (see Case 6) and are also seen in hypertension and in AD, affecting around a fifth of patients with this condition. The diagnostic and prognostic characteristics of BMBs are uncertain and thus their presence can give rise to clinical dilemmas as illustrated in the current case (see answer to Question 3).

In a population-based cross-sectional sample of 1062 people aged 60 years and older without dementia, BMBs were more prevalent among users of antiplatelet drugs (adjusted odds ratio 1.71, 95% CI 1.2–2.4). However, these findings do not necessarily indicate that patients with BMBs are at increased risk of bleeding when treated with antiplatelet drugs since BMBs may be related to the underlying vascular disease.

Recently, Lovelock *et al.* (2010) undertook a pooled analysis of 3817 patients with ischaemic stroke or TIA and 1460 patients with ICH, and found an excess of BMBs in warfarin-associated ICH that was not found in patients who had an ischaemic stroke or TIA while on warfarin. These preliminary data indicate that warfarin may be hazardous in patients with BMBs. Similar but weaker associations between BMB frequency and antiplatelet-associated ICH were also seen, but significant heterogeneity between cohorts means that these results should be interpreted with caution. Available prospective data are few but support the hypothesis that the presence of BMBs increases the risk of future ICH with antithrombotic drug use. More prospective data on the safety of antithrombotic drugs in patients with microbleeds are urgently required, but at present antithrombotic treatment should not be withheld in situations where there is established overall benefit. Decisions regarding antithrombotic

treatment are particularly difficult in CAA where there are high risks of both ischaemic and haemorrhagic strokes (see Case 6).

3. Would you warfarinize this patient?

Deciding whether or not to give anticoagulation is not straightforward.

In the setting of ischaemic stroke accompanied by PAF, warfarin would usually
be the secondary preventative treatment of choice. However, the risks and benefits
of warfarin should always be carefully considered on an individual patient basis (see
Case 22). Warfarin was not given to the current patient because of the combination
of Crohn's disease, anaemia, and the microhaemorrhages seen on the MRI. She was
referred to cardiology for consideration of antiarrythmic treatment. However, at
present, there is little evidence to suggest that treatment to maintain sinus rhythm
is more effective in preventing stroke than rate control of AF, and anticoagulation
is recommended in both strategies (see Case 22).

Further reading

Lovelock CE, Cordonnier C, Naka H, *et al.* (2010). Antithrombotic drug use, cerebral
microbleeds, and intracerebral hemorrhage: a systematic review of published and
unpublished studies. *Stroke*; **41**: 1222–8.

Thijs V, Lemmens R, Schoofs C, *et al.* (2010). Microbleeds and the risk of recurrent stroke.
Stroke; **41**: 2005–9.

Vernooij MW, Haag MD, van der Lugt A, *et al.* (2009). Use of antithrombotic drugs and the
presence of cerebral microbleeds: the Rotterdam Scan Study. *Arch Neurol*; **66**: 714–20.

Case 42

A 67-year-old man was taken to the accident and emergency department. His wife had found him lying on the floor in the living room. He was initially unconscious, but within the next 15 minutes woke up, and appeared restless and confused. He had a right hemiparesis and also had word-finding difficulties. The patient had a history of hypertension, and he was on warfarin for PAF. This had been started 6 months previously when he had had a left MCA infarction from which he had made a good recovery, although he still had some persisting mild right-sided weakness. There was no history of other medical problems. The patient's medication included antihypertensives and a statin in addition to warfarin.

Questions

1. What is your differential diagnosis?
2. How would you investigate this patient?
3. How would you treat the patient?

Answers

1. What is your differential diagnosis?

The patient's symptoms suggest involvement of the left MCA territory, i.e. the same territory that was affected in his previous stroke. The differential diagnosis includes the following:

◆ A further ischaemic stroke due to cardioembolism, although it would be unusual for this to affect the same territory as previously. Furthermore, MCA infarcts only very rarely produce loss of consciousness.

◆ A cerebral haemorrhage promoted by hypertension and warfarin.

◆ A secondary generalized seizure originating from the area damaged by the previous stroke. This would explain the patient's collapse, loss of consciousness, and confusion. His right-sided weakness and dysphasia would then be due to Todd's paresis.

2. How would you investigate this patient?

The patient requires urgent brain imaging because he has a neurological deficit and he is on warfarin. A cerebral haemorrhage needs to be excluded. Depending on the imaging modality (CT or MRI) and on the time since event, the scan might also show new ischaemic changes. In the current patient, a CT brain scan showed no haemorrhage but only the established infarction from 6 months earlier. The patient should also have blood tests, including an INR to see if his anticoagulation is adequate, and a full blood count, electrolytes, and blood sugar to look for underlying infection or a metabolic derangement that might have caused a seizure. Equally, cardiac arrhythmias can cause a collapse, and associated cerebral hypoxia may cause a seizure. Therefore the patient should also have an ECG and, if felt appropriate, may require longer ECG monitoring. In the current patient, the INR was in the therapeutic range, the other blood tests were normal, and the ECG showed atrial fibrillation as the only abnormality.

The patient was kept in hospital overnight. He had fully recovered by the next morning, but then had a witnessed generalized seizure which again was followed by a right hemiparesis. This confirmed the suspected diagnosis of seizure and Todd's paresis, with the most likely underlying cause for the seizure being his previous stroke.

Todd's paralysis was first described in detail by Robert Todd in the late nineteenth century. He observed transient paralysis after epileptic seizures and assumed that this was due to 'a state of depression or exhaustion, not only in the parts primarily affected, but in parts of the brain connected with them'. The phenomenon of post-epileptic paralysis has been described and studied in more detail since then, but the pathophysiology of this phenomenon, and whether it is due to depressed neuronal metabolism or to inhibition of motor centres, remains uncertain. However, clinically it is important to be aware of this phenomenon as it may mimic other conditions (e.g. cerebrovascular events, as in the current case).

3. How would you treat the patient?

About 10% of patients have a seizure after a stroke, and about a third of those (3% absolute number) develop post-stroke epilepsy. Seizures are divided into early and late onset, with the arbitrary cut-off for this classification being 2 weeks. It is unclear which patients are at risk of developing seizures after a stroke. Generally the risk after a cerebral haemorrhage is thought to be higher than that after an ischaemic event. Strokes with cortical involvement have a higher risk than subcortical lesions, and the larger the area of cortex that is involved, the higher the risk of having a seizure. Patients with late-onset seizures seem to have a higher risk of recurrence than patients with early-onset seizures. Some studies report that the risk of recurrence in patients with late-onset seizures is as high as 90%. This is most likely due to the presence of a permanent lesion which causes persistent changes in neuronal excitability. Gliotic scarring is thought to be the culprit for late-onset seizures.

Our patient has had late-onset seizures and is at a high risk of recurrent fits. Given that these carry a risk of injury and death, in particular as the patient is also on warfarin and therefore at an increased risk of haemorrhage if he has an injury, he should be started on anticonvulsant therapy. As post-stroke seizures are of focal onset, the drugs of choice according to the SANAD study are carbamazepine or lamotrigine. The efficacy of both drugs is similar. The advantages of lamotrigine are its better side-effect profile and its lack of interaction with warfarin. However, it takes a long time to titrate up to a therapeutic dose. A further drug to consider may be levetiracetam, which also has only a few drug interactions, is tolerated well, and can be titrated up more quickly. Generally, post-stroke seizures respond well to anticonvulsant therapy, with 88% of patients being well controlled on mono-therapy. In addition to anticonvulsant medication, the patient and his family should be advised about driving (see Case 23) and avoiding hazardous situations, and they should be offered further counselling.

Further reading

Binder DK (2004). A history of Todd and his paralysis. *Neurosurgery*; **54**: 480–7.

Marson AG, Al-Kharusi AM, Alwaidh M, *et al.* (2007). The SANAD study of effectiveness of carbamazepine, gabapentin, lamotrigine, oxcarbazepine, or topiramate for treatment of partial epilepsy: an unblinded randomised controlled trial. *Lancet*; **369**: 1000–15.

Myint PK, Staufenberg EFA, Sabanathan K (2006). Post-stroke seizure and post-stroke epilepsy. *Postgrad Med J*; **82**: 568–72.

Silverman IE, Restrepo L, Mathews GC (2002). Poststroke seizures. *Arch Neurol*; **59**: 195–202.

Case 43

Case 43.A

A 78-year-old woman was admitted with confusion and odd behaviour that had developed over the preceding day. There was a history of stroke causing left-sided weakness 2 years previously, from which she had made a good recovery, AF, and hypertension. Medication included amlodipine, aspirin, simvastatin, and digoxin. She lived alone in warden-controlled accommodation. Her son reported some cognitive deterioration over the last 2 years such that she required some help with finances and shopping.

Examination was limited because of her agitated state: she was unable to follow commands and was very distractible, with poor concentration. Pulse was 90bpm in AF and blood pressure was 170/80mm Hg. Cranial nerves appeared normal and there was probable mild right upper limb weakness and an extensor right plantar response. Her speech was confused and much of it was incomprehensible; formal assessment was not possible. She was agitated, especially in the evenings and at night, and was combative when interacting with staff. On occasions, she adopted a fetal position, refusing any contact.

Investigations showed the following:

- WCC 10.2; CRP 4
- Blood glucose, creatinine and electrolytes, and liver and thyroid function tests all normal
- Urinalysis: negative
- ECG: AF, no other significant abnormalities
- CXR: clear
- CT brain is shown in Fig. 43.1

Case 43.B

An 85-year-old woman was admitted with worsening confusion, slurred speech, and agitation. Her son reported some possible left facial weakness. There was a past history of osteoarthritis, cognitive impairment, and physical decline over the last few years and TIA 6 months previously. Her son was certain that there had been an acute decline in her cognitive function. She was usually mobile with a frame, and she lived with her elderly husband and son. On examination, pulse was regular at 90bpm and blood pressure was elevated at 210/100mmHg; oxygen saturations were 96% on air. She was agitated and resistant to examination, but there was evidence of upper motor neuron left facial weakness and unsafe swallow, and her speech was incoherent. During admission, she repeatedly pulled out cannulae and was agitated, particularly in the evenings.

Investigations showed the following:

- Routine bloods were unremarkable
- MRI brain is shown in Fig. 43.2

Questions

1. What syndrome do these cases illustrate?
2. What is the most likely cause in patients A and B? What are the risk factors present in each case that predispose to the syndrome in Question 1?
3. What is the prognosis from a cognitive perspective?

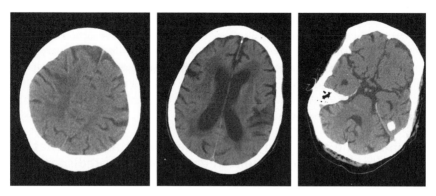

Fig. 43.1 CT brain for patient A.

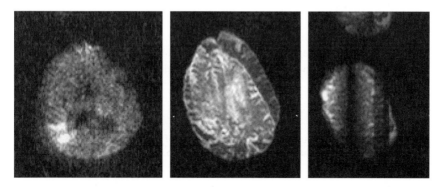

Fig. 43.2 DWI brain for patient B.

Answers

1. What syndrome do these cases illustrate?

These cases illustrate the syndrome of delirium. Criteria for delirium are described in DSM-IV (see Table 43.1).

Patients with delirium are often agitated, although some may be unusually sleepy. Attention deficits are prominent, with the patient showing poor concentration and distractibility. Speech is muddled with evidence of disordered thinking. There is fluctuation in mental state with a tendency for confusion to become more obvious in the evenings and at night, such that patients may appear normal on the morning ward round but be sufficiently disturbed to require sedation at night. Delirium is highly prevalent in elderly general medical inpatients and after surgery, especially for hip fracture, and associated factors include increasing age, background cognitive impairment, severity of illness, comorbidity, and environmental characteristics. It is associated with increased mortality and length of stay, institutionalization, and risk of dementia in the medium and longer term.

2. What is the most likely cause in patients A and B? What are the risk factors present in each case that predispose to the syndrome in Question 1?

The most likely cause of delirium in patients A and B is a stroke.

The investigations in both patient A and patient B show no evidence of sepsis to explain a delirium. In patient A, the presence of right-sided weakness and incomprehensible speech suggests a left hemisphere ischaemic event (since no bleed was seen on the CT), which was probably cortical. The risk factors for delirium in this patient include older age, comorbidity (hypertension, AF, previous stroke), pre-existing cognitive impairment, polypharmacy, and acute stroke. The CT shows

Table 43.1 DSM-IV criteria for delirium

---

1. **Disturbance of consciousness (i.e. reduced clarity of awareness of the environment) with reduced ability to focus, sustain, or shift attention**

2. **Change in cognition** (e.g. memory deficit, disorientation, language disturbance, and perceptual disturbance) that is not better accounted for by a pre-existing, established, or evolving dementia

3. **Development over a short period of time** (usually hours to days) and disturbance **tends to fluctuate** during the course of the day

4. **Evidence from the history, physical examination, or laboratory findings that the disturbance**:
   - is caused by the direct physiological consequences of a **general medical condition**
   - developed during substance intoxication
   - was aetiologically related to the use of **medication**
   - developed during, or shortly after, **a withdrawal syndrome**
   - was caused by an unknown precipitant (**not otherwise specified)**

---

extensive atrophy. In patient B, there was a history of possible focal weakness, a past history of TIA, and a background of cognitive impairment. The DWI scan, although degraded by movement artefact, shows an acute right hemisphere lesion. Delirium is relatively common after stroke (~24%) and may be the presenting feature, as in the above cases. The risk factors for stroke-associated delirium are similar to those for delirium in general but with the addition of stroke-related factors such as greater lesion size and left-sided lesions.

3. What is the prognosis from a cognitive perspective?

The prognosis is poor regarding cognitive outcome.

Acute confusion in stroke is predictive of post-stroke dementia. In a systematic review and meta-analysis of stroke-related dementia, acute confusion in the first few days after stroke was associated with an odds ratio (OR) of around 6 for the development of dementia at 6 months compared with patients without acute confusion. This is similar to the OR for the development of dementia after delirium during admissions for an acute general medical condition (OR of 5 for dementia at 3 years).

Patient A gradually improved over the next week and it became apparent that she had receptive and expressive dysphasia. Although her speech improved to some extent and she had no limb weakness, she required help with activities of daily living and was ultimately discharged to a care home. In patient B, the delirium was severe and continued for the next few weeks, requiring use of antipsychotics for the management of disturbed behaviour. The behaviour eventually normalized but the patient was left with significant cognitive impairment consistent with dementia. She returned home to live with her family with support from professional carers visiting daily.

Further reading

Caeiro L, Ferro JM, Albuquerque R, Figueira ML (2004). Delirium in the first days of acute stroke. *J Neurol*; **251**: 171–8.

Ferro JM, Caeiro L, Verdelho A (2002). Delirium in acute stroke. *Curr Opin Neurol*; **15**: 51–5.

Henon H, Lebert F, Durieu I, *et al.* (1999). Confusional state in stroke: relation to preexisting dementia, patient characteristics, and outcome. *Stroke*; **30**: 773–9.

Oldenbeuving AW, de Kort PL, Jansen BP, Algra A, Kappelle LJ, Roks G (2011). Delirium in the acute phase after stroke: incidence, risk factors, and outcome. *Neurology*; **76**: 993–9.

Pendlebury ST, Rothwell PM (2009). Prevalence, incidence, and factors associated with pre-stroke and post-stroke dementia: a systematic review and meta-analysis. *Lancet Neurol*; **8**: 1006–18.

Siddiqi N, House AO, Holmes JD (2006). Occurrence and outcome of delirium in medical in-patients: a systematic literature review. *Age Ageing*; **35**: 350–64.

Case 44

Case 44.A

A 46-year-old woman was referred to the TIA clinic. She had a long history of migraine, with attacks occurring approximately four times per year. She usually had no aura, apart from one episode of dysphasia associated with a migraine attack 13 years earlier. Two weeks prior to her clinic attendance she had developed her usual migraine headache, which 2 hours later was followed by a sudden onset of dysarthria. She described that she had found it difficult to move her tongue and jaw. This persisted until the next morning. She had also been aware of pins and needles affecting the right side of her face, but this only lasted for a few seconds. The patient had an MRI scan of her brain (Fig. 44.1).

Case 44.B

A 48-year-old woman presented to the neurology clinic with a history of generalized headache which had been present on and off for the past 10 years and became worse when she was stressed. Recently the headaches had become more frequent, which prompted the neurology referral and an MRI brain scan (Fig. 44.2). The patient was otherwise well, with no medical problems in the past. She was on no medication apart from co-codamol for the headache.

Questions

1. What do the MRI scans show?
2. How do these lesions most commonly present?
3. Which part of the history will most commonly differ between patients with the scan appearance in Fig. 44.1 and the scan appearance in Fig. 44.2?
4. When and how should these lesions be treated?

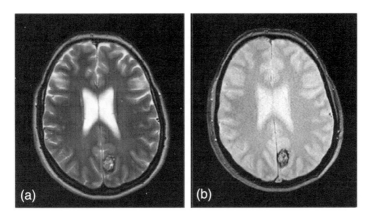

Fig. 44.1 MRI brain. Axial T2-weighted image (a), and GRE (b).

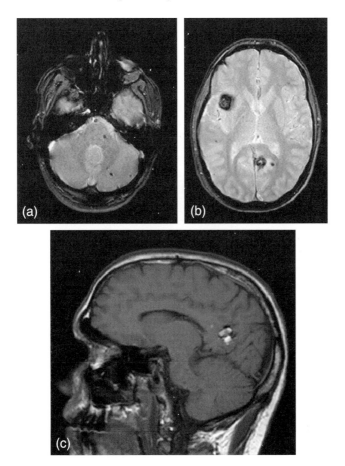

Fig. 44.2 MRI brain scan. Axial GRE sequences ((a), (b)) and sagittal T1-weighted image (c).

Answers

1. What do the MRI scans show?

The MRI scan in Fig. 44.1 shows a single cavernous haemangioma (cavernoma) in the left parieto-occipital lobe. The cavernoma shows the typical appearance of mixed signal intensity in the centre, which represents blood products of different ages and calcification. The cavernoma is surrounded by a black ring of haemosiderin. This is more obvious on GRE (Fig. 44.1(b)) than on a standard T2-weighted image (Fig 41.1(a)) because of the greater sensitivity of this sequence to magnetic susceptibility effects. Cavernomas are not usually associated with oedema or mass effect, and they do not usually show up on angiography. MRI brain with GRE is the most sensitive imaging method to show cavernomas, as this will reveal blood breakdown products of different ages and has a higher resolution than CT. The MRI scan in Fig. 44.2 shows multiple cavernomas. Figures 44.2(a) and 44.2(b) are axial gradient echo images. They show multiple microhaemorrhages in the cerebellum, which most likely represent small cavernomas, and two larger cavernomas in the right basal ganglia and the left medial occipital lobe. The sagittal T1-weighted image (Fig.44.2(c)) shows the left occipital cavernoma also visible in Fig. 44.2(b). A mixed intensity signal within a cavernoma can indicate blood products of different ages. However, in this patient the high signal indicates calcification, as the appearance of the lesion had not changed over 2 years and calcification can have high signal on T1-weighted images.

2. How do these lesions most commonly present?

Cavernomas are vascular malformations that consist of enlarged capillary-like vessels without intervening parenchyma. Macroscopically they are well circumscribed and have a 'mulberry-like' appearance. Their incidence in the general population is 0.1–0.9%. They occur with similar frequency in men and women, although there seems to be a slight female preponderance for multiple cavernomas.

Cavernomas can be clinically silent. Approximately 20% of cavernomas are diagnosed as an incidental finding on brain imaging done for other reasons, as in patient B. Epileptic seizures are the most common clinical presentation. They occur in 40–50% of patients, and seizure control can often be difficult. Headache has been described in 6–52% of patients. However, this is a frequent symptom also in the general population, and it is difficult to know if the reported headache really is due to the cavernoma. Ten to forty per cent of patients present with a focal neurological deficit. This can be due to change in lesion size, haemorrhage, thrombosis, or peri-lesional iron deposition. The deficit may be permanent or fluctuate. Sometimes the clinical course may mimic multiple sclerosis. Finally, 13–56% of cavernomas present with a symptomatic haemorrhage.

3. Which part of the history will most commonly differ between patients with the scan appearance in Fig. 44.1 and the scan appearance in Fig. 44.2?

Figure 44.1 shows a single cavernoma. These are usually sporadic. Figure 44.2 shows multiple cavernomas. Patients with multiple lesions usually have a hereditary form of cavernomatosis, and therefore will often have a family history of this disorder or associated symptoms, for example a family history of epilepsy or early stroke and brain haemorrhages. Mutations at three loci (*CCM1*, *CCM2*, and *CCM3*) have now been identified for familial forms of cavernous malformations. All of these are autosomal dominant. Clinical penetrance is incomplete (60–80%), with penetrance for having lesions on neuroimaging being much higher, although not quite 100%.

4. When and how should these lesions be treated?

Management of cavernomas is usually conservative. Surgery is generally reserved for patients with intractable seizures and progressive focal symptoms, and to reduce the risk of haemorrhage. The quoted risk of haemorrhage from a cavernoma varies between studies, but is generally estimated to be 0.1–2.5% per lesion per year. It is probably higher if there has been a previous haemorrhage. Therefore surgery will be indicated in patients with recurrent haemorrhage. In some cases, it may also be considered for young patients with easily accessible single lesions, as they have a high cumulative risk of haemorrhage. The decision for surgical intervention will also depend on the location of the cavernoma. Lesions in non-eloquent cortex can be removed with less risk than lesions in eloquent areas, or deep lesions in the basal ganglia or brainstem. Radiosurgical intervention may be an alternative for some of the deep-seated lesions, but currently its benefit is still controversial.

Patient A continued to have severe and frequent headaches after her intial presentation to the clinic. She also developed an associated visual disturbance. Because there was evidence of recent haemorrhage on the scan, and as the location of the cavernoma was appropriate to cause the patient's visual symptoms, eventually the decision was made to proceed to stereotactic removal of the cavernoma. The patient tolerated this well, and only had a transient visual field defect after the surgery. Removal of the cavernoma was complete, and the headache subsequently improved markedly.

Further reading

Labauge P, Denier C, Bergametti F, Tournier-Lasserve E (2007). Genetics of cavernous angiomas. *Lancet Neurol*; **6**: 237–44.

Metellus P, Kharkar S, Lin D, Kapoor S, Rigamonti D (2008). Cerebral cavernous malformations and developmental venous anomalies. In: Caplan LR (ed.), *Uncommon causes of stroke* (2nd edn). Cambridge: Cambridge University Press: 189–219.

Case 45

Case 45.A

An 81-year-old right-handed woman had sudden onset of right hand weakness and tingling at 10.00 which lasted for 15 minutes and then resolved completely. She experienced four further similar episodes each lasting for 15–20 minutes over the next few hours. At 18.30 she had yet another episode of right arm and leg weakness and slurred speech which persisted. She called her GP who arranged admission to hospital.

Investigations showed the following:

- ◆ ECG: sinus rhythm
- ◆ Carotid Doppler: no significant stenosis
- ◆ CT brain is shown in Fig. 45.1.

Case 45.B

A 72-year-old man got up at 04.00 to use the bathroom, and found that his left arm and left leg were weak and numb. His wife noticed that his face was drooping on the left and that his speech was slurred. His symptoms lasted for 20 minutes and then resolved but recurred after 30 minutes with more severe weakness, this time lasting for 15 minutes. An ambulance was called at 05.00. He had a further episode in the ambulance and another two in the emergency department, each resolving within 15 minutes.

On examination in the emergency department during an episode of weakness, the pulse was 80bpm regular, blood pressure was 245/84mmHg, and left arm and leg tone were flaccid with power of 4/5 in the left arm and 2/5 in the left leg.

Investigations showed the following:

- ◆ ECG: sinus rhythm, left ventricular hypertrophy
- ◆ Carotid Dopplers: normal
- ◆ CT brain: normal

The patient was discharged on aspirin, a statin, and antihypertensive therapy but 2 days later at 05:00 he had sudden-onset left-sided weakness and felt 'drunk'. He returned to the emergency department immediately, and on examination had left-sided weakness and left limb ataxia (ataxic hemiparesis). A further CT brain scan showed no change.

Case 45.C

An 89-year-old right-handed man had sudden right arm weakness at 10.00 whilst holding a cup of coffee. The symptoms resolved after a few minutes. There was a further episode of right hand weakness at 13.00, and at 16.00 he developed right leg weakness such that he was unable to get out of his chair. Both episodes resolved within minutes. At 20.00, he experienced sudden-onset right arm and leg weakness, which persisted. Overnight, he got up to go to the toilet and felt that his balance was poor.

He called his GP the next morning and was admitted with an NIH Stroke Score (NIHSS) of 6. The diagnosis was felt to be possible ataxic hemiparesis or pure motor lacunar stroke.

MRI brain (DWI) is shown in Fig. 45.2.

Questions .

1. What clinical syndrome do these three cases illustrate?
2. What is the mechanism of this condition?

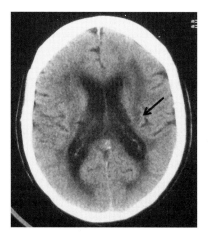

Fig. 45.1 CT brain of patient A shows widespread small vessel disease. There is also a lacunar infarct in the deep periventricular white matter (arrow).

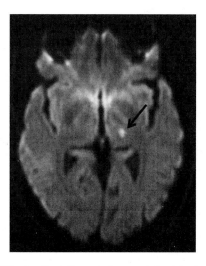

Fig. 45.2 MRI brain (DWI) of patient C: acute lacunar infarct in the left thalamus (arrow).

Answers

1. What clinical syndrome do these three cases illustrate?

These cases are all examples of capsular warning syndrome preceding lacunar infarction.

The capsular warning syndrome has a rather characteristic pattern in which there is a cluster of TIAs, consisting typically of weakness down the whole of one side of the body without any cognitive or language deficit (i.e. pure motor lacunar TIAs). These may be followed within hours or days by a lacunar infarct in the internal capsule.

The vast majority of lacunar stroke syndromes are caused by ischaemia rather than haemorrhage. Most ischaemic lacunar strokes are the result of a small deep, not cortical, infarct. These small deep infarcts are usually located within the distribution of a small perforating artery. More than 20 lacunar syndromes have been described. Five have been validated as being highly predictive for the presence of lacunes radiologically:

- pure motor hemiparesis
- pure sensory stroke
- ataxic hemiparesis
- sensorimotor stroke
- dysarthria–clumsy hand syndrome.

The presence of one of the above five syndromes has a positive predictive value of 87–90% for detecting a radiological lacune, although some clinical syndromes are more predictive than others. Preceding TIAs and non-sudden onset may increase the positive predictive value. Predicted infarct locations in relation to clinical manifestations are shown in Table 45.1.

2. What is the mechanism of this condition?

Presumably capsular warning syndrome is caused by intermittent closure of a single lenticulostriate or other perforating artery, followed by complete occlusion.

The aetiology of lacunar stroke is unclear. A systematic review of 19 cohort studies involving 5864 patients with ischaemic stroke found that those who had a lacunar infarct as the index event were more likely to have recurrence of lacunar stroke than non-lacunar stroke. This suggests that lacunar strokes may represent a different form of arteriopathy from other ischaemic stroke subtypes. Rates of carotid stenosis and risk factors for cardioembolism are much lower in patients with lacunes than in patients with cortical infarcts, and may be similar to that of asymptomatic elderly populations. It also appears that patients with lacunar infarcts more often have milder degrees of carotid stenosis than those with cortical infarcts, although ipsilateral carotid stenosis appears to be more common than contralateral stenosis, supporting a possible causal role for large vessel disease.

Several mechanisms have been proposed for occlusion of small penetrator branches in lacunar stroke:

- lipohyalinosis of the penetrating arteries, particularly in smaller infarcts (3–7mm in diameter)

Table 45.1 Predicted infarct locations

Lacunar syndrome	Location	Clinical findings	Positive predictive value
Pure motor hemiparesis	Internal capsule; corona radiata; basal pons; medial medulla	Unilateral paralysis of face, arm, and leg; no sensory signs; dysarthria and dysphagia may be present	52–85%
Pure sensory syndrome	Thalamus; pontine tegmentum; corona radiata	Unilateral numbness of face, arm, and leg without motor deficit	95–100%
Ataxic hemiparesis	Internal capsule; corona radiata; basal pons; thalamus	Unilateral weakness and limb ataxia	59–95%
Sensorimotor syndrome	Thalamocapsular; maybe basal pons or lateral medulla	Hemiparesis or hemiplegia of face; arm and leg with ipsilateral sensory impairment	51–87%
Dysarthria–clumsy hand syndrome	Basal pons; internal capsule; corona radiata	Unilateral facial weakness; dysarthria and dysphagia with mild hand weakness and clumsiness	About 96%

- atheroma at the origin of the penetrating arteries
- small emboli.

There is pathological evidence to support the first two of the above mechanisms which are thought to be a consequence of systemic hypertension. The third mechanism is supported by case reports of lacunes in patients with high-risk cardiac sources for emboli or following cardiac angiography.

Other mechanisms which have been proposed to account for lacunar infarcts include failure of the arteriolar endothelium and the blood–brain barrier. Blood–brain barrier permeability is thought to allow extravasation of blood components into the vessel wall, resulting in damage to the vessel wall, perivascular neurons, and glia.

Further reading

Boiten J, Lodder J (1991). Lacunar infarcts: pathogenesis and validity of the clinical syndromes. *Stroke*; **22**: 1374–8.

Donnan GA, O'Malley RN, Quang L, Hurley S, Bladin PF (1993). The capsular warning syndrome: pathogenesis and clinical features. *Neurology*; **43**: 957–62.

Gan R, Sacco RL, Kargman DE, *et al.* (1997). Testing the validity of the lacunar hypothesis: the Northern Manhattan Stroke Study experience. *Neurology*; **48**: 1204–11.

Gorman MJ, Dafer R, Levine SR (1998). Ataxic hemiparesis: critical appraisal of a lacunar syndrome. *Stroke*; **29**: 2549.

Hervé D, Gautier-Bertrand M, Labreuche J, *et al.* (2004). Predictive values of lacunar transient ischemic attacks. *Stroke*; **35**: 1430–5.

Melo TP, Bogousslavsky J, van Melle G, Regli F (1992). Pure motor stroke: a reappraisal. *Neurology*; **42**: 789–95.

Moulin T, Bogousslavsky J, Chopard JL, *et al.* (1995). Vascular ataxic hemiparesis: a re-evaluation. *J Neurol Neurosurg Psychiatry*; **58**: 422–7.

Prabhakaram S, Krakauer JW (2006). Multiple reversible episodes of subcortical ischaemic following postcoital middle cerebral artery dissection. *Arch Neurol*; **63**: 891–3.

Toni D, Del Duca R, Fiorelli M, *et al.* (1994). Pure motor hemiparesis and sensorimotor stroke. Accuracy of very early clinical diagnosis of lacunar strokes. *Stroke*; **25**: 92–6.

Wardlaw JM, Doubal F, Armitage P, *et al.* (2009). Lacunar stroke is associated with diffuse blood–brain barrier dysfunction. *Ann Neurol*; **65**: 194–202.

Case 46

A 79-year-old man presented to the TIA clinic with sudden onset of left upper limb and left facial numbness and weakness and mildly slurred speech that had resolved after half an hour. There was a history of abdominal aortic aneurysm repair, hypertension, and AF and he was taking warfarin. The CT brain is shown in Fig. 46.1.

Questions

1. What is the diagnosis? What are the risk factors for this condition? How long ago did this happen?
2. How would you manage this case?

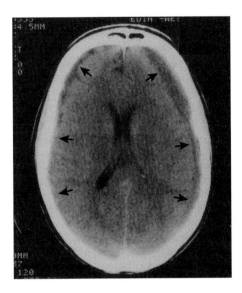

Fig. 46.1 CT brain.

Answers

1. What is the diagnosis? What are the risk factors for this condition? How long ago did this happen?

The diagnosis is bilateral subdural haematomas.

Subdural haematoma (SDH) may present with sudden-onset transient focal neurological deficit although there is often a preceding history of confusion, headache, or drowsiness. The insidious onset of headache, light-headedness, cognitive impairment, apathy, somnolence, and occasionally seizures may occur as a consequence of chronic SDH, and symptoms may not become evident until weeks after the initial injury. Global deficits such as disturbance of consciousness are more common than focal deficits after SDH.

Focal deficits may be either ipsilateral or contralateral to the side of the SDH. Contralateral hemiparesis can occur as a result of direct compression of cortex underlying the haematoma, whereas ipsilateral hemiparesis can occur with lateral displacement of the midbrain caused by the mass effect of the haematoma. Such midbrain displacement results in compression of the contralateral cerebral peduncle against the free edge of the tentorium.

SDH is more common in the elderly, alcoholics, and those taking anticoagulants, and only about 50% of patients recall having had a head injury or a fall. Haemorrhage occurs secondary to tearing of the bridging veins that drain from the surface of the brain to the dural sinuses, and blood accumulates in the space between the arachnoid membranes and dura across which the vessels traverse. Venous bleeding usually stops owing to rising intracranial pressure or direct compression by the clot itself. Arterial rupture can also result in SDH, and this source accounts for approximately 20–30% of SDH cases.

The SDH in Fig. 46.1 is at least 21 days old since the blood is hypodense. The age of an SDH can be determined from its appearance on CT. Acutely; the CT shows an area of hyperdensity in the subdural space, ipsilateral sulcal effacement, and sometimes ventricular shift and distortion. Between 7 and 21 days after onset, the blood becomes isointense and can easily be missed, especially if there are bilateral haematomas resulting in a symmetrical appearance (Fig. 46.2). After 21 days the haematoma becomes hypodense. Sometimes blood of varying ages may be seen (Fig. 46.3). MRI is more sensitive than CT at demonstrating SDH, particularly beyond the acute stage and where the volume of subdural bleeding is small.

Following the initial meningeal trauma and development of SDH, dural collagen synthesis is induced and fibroblasts spread over the inner surface of the dura to form a thick outer membrane. Over the next couple of weeks, a thinner inner membrane develops, resulting in complete encapsulation of the clot. Over time, a chronic SDH may liquefy to form a hygroma (Fig. 46.4) and the membranes may calcify. More than half of all SDHs liquefy and may enlarge. Larger initial clot size appears to be related to a greater likelihood of subsequent expansion. At any time, the haematoma may expand secondary to recurrent bleeding ('acute-on-chronic' SDH) or from osmotic draw of water into the hygroma owing to its high protein content.

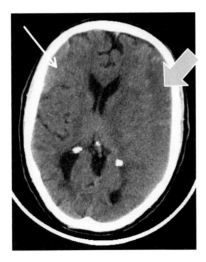

Fig. 46.2 This patient has bilateral SDHs. The right frontal haematoma is subacute (white arrow); blood is still visible as hyperdense. The haematoma over the left hemsiphere is older and almost isointense with brain tissue (filled grey arrow).

Thalamic lesions and secondary brainstem injury may develop as a consequence of the mass effect produced by a large SDH.

2. How would you manage this case?

Coexistent anticoagulation in patients with either traumatic or spontaneous SDH is not uncommon and must be reversed before surgical intervention. Ideally, anticoagulation should also be reversed for those patients who are managed non-operatively. However, the potential benefit of reversing anticoagulation (a reduced risk of haematoma enlargement) must be weighed against the risk related to the underlying need for anticoagulation in this group (e.g. AF, mechanical heart valve).

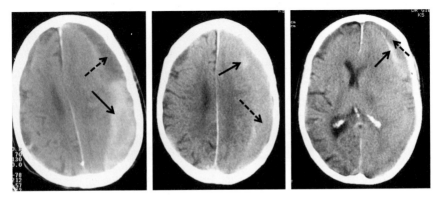

Fig. 46.3 Acute-on-chronic SDH showing hyperdense blood on a background of hypodense and isointense blood (arrows).

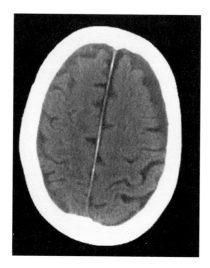

Fig. 46.4 Subdural hygroma.

Acute symptomatic SDH is a neurological emergency that often requires surgical treatment to prevent irreversible brain injury and death caused by haematoma expansion, elevated intracranial pressure, and brain herniation.

There are few data available to guide management of chronic SDH. For patients with chronic SDH and the potential for recovery, surgical evacuation of the haematoma should be considered if there is evidence of moderate to severe cognitive impairment or progressive neurological deterioration, or if there is clot thickness ≥10 mm or significant midline shift (Fig. 46.5).

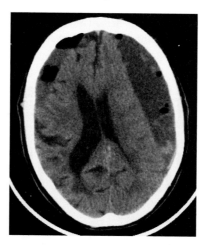

Fig. 46.5 Bilateral SDH, left larger than right. The haematoma on the left has caused compression of the left lateral ventricle and midline shift. The dark areas within the haematoma are air, which are a sign that there has been recent surgical drainage of the haematoma with subsequent re-collection of fluid.

Further reading

Adhiyaman V, Asghar M, Ganeshram KN, Bhowmick BK (2002). Chronic subdural haematoma in the elderly. *Postgrad Med J*; **78**: 71–5.

Chen JC, Levy ML (2000). Causes, epidemiology, and risk factors of chronic subdural hematoma. *Neurosurg Clin N Am*; **11**: 399–406.

Downer JJ, Pretorius PM (2009). Symmetry in computed tomography of the brain: the pitfalls. *Clin Radiol*; **64**: 298–306.

Iantosca MR, Simon RH (2000). Chronic subdural hematoma in adult and elderly patients. *Neurosurg Clin N Am*; **11**: 447–54.

Moster ML, Johnston DE, Reinmuth OM (1983). Chronic subdural haematoma with transient neurological deficits: a review of 15 cases. *Ann Neurol*; **14**: 539–42.

Udstuen GJ, Claar JM (2001). Imaging of acute head injury in the adult. *Semin Ultrasound CT MR*; **22**: 135–47.

Case 47

An 84-year-old woman was referred by her GP to the TIA clinic with an episode of visual disturbance. She reported that a week previously, she had transiently lost the vision in her right eye. The day before she was seen in the clinic she had had a 5 minute episode of 'odd speech' and a 'twisted mouth' seen by her husband. One month before she had been discharged following a prolonged admission with an infected right hip replacement following hip surgery some months previously. She had lost 2 stone in weight whilst being unwell, but this had stabilized recently. Over the 3 weeks prior to coming to the TIA clinic, she had felt less well again with malaise and hot flushes. There was a past history of mild hypertension but nothing else.

On examination, she looked pale with a temperature of 38.2°C, pulse of 96bpm regular, and blood pressure 108/80mmHg. There was an ejection systolic murmur radiating to the neck and a pan systolic murmur at the apex. There was also thought to be a quiet early diastolic murmur. Neurological examination revealed mild right facial weakness but normal limb power. The skin over the right hip felt warm.

Investigations showed the following:

- Hb 10.2; WCC 26.03; platelets 590; ESR 24; CRP 201
- Na 123; K 3.9; Cr 120; Ca 2.58; albumin 44; bilirubin 8; alanine aminotransferase (ALT) 37; AlkP 426; GGT 180
- CXR: enlarged heart, clear lungs
- Left hip X-ray: hip replacement, no other abnormality
- CT brain showed an infarct in the right MCA territory.

Questions

1. What is the likely underlying diagnosis?
2. What are the possible causes of focal neurological deficits in this condition?
3. What further investigations would you request?
4. How would you manage this condition?

Answers

1. What is the likely underlying diagnosis?

The CT brain shows a probable right hemispheric infarct, and the most likely unifying diagnosis is infective endocarditis (IE).

This woman has developed symptoms consistent with transient ischaemia affecting the right eye followed by a further episode of ischaemia affecting the left hemisphere. The presence of two separate episodes affecting different vascular territories suggests the presence of a cardioembolic source (see Cases 4 and 37). The recent history of an infected hip replacement and malaise together with the pyrexia, cardiac murmurs, and elevated inflammatory markers makes IE the most likely underlying diagnosis. This case illustrates the fact that endocarditis may present with focal cerebral ischaemia and that such symptoms may be transient or leave only mild residual deficits. It should always be considered in patients with a history of recent sepsis, especially skin or bone/joint infection, and in intravenous drug abusers or those who are systemically unwell.

The diagnosis of IE is straightforward in patients with classic clinical (Oslerian) features including positive blood cultures, active valvulitis, peripheral emboli, and immunological vascular phenomena. However, classic features may be absent in other patients, particularly in hyper-acute disease (e.g. in intravenous drug users with *Staphylococcus aureus* infection of right-sided heart valves). Immunological vascular phenomena are more common in subacute IE.

The variability in clinical presentation prompted the development of the Duke criteria by Durack and colleagues in 1994 which stratified patients with suspected IE into three categories: 'definite' cases, identified either clinically or pathologically (surgery or autopsy), 'possible' cases, and 'rejected' cases (no pathological evidence of IE at autopsy or surgery, rapid resolution of the clinical syndrome with either no treatment or short-term antibiotic therapy, or a firm alternative diagnosis). The Duke criteria have subsequently been modified (see Tables 47.1 and 47.2).

2. What are the possible causes of focal neurological deficits in this condition?

The causes of focal neurological deficits in infective endocarditis are:

- ischaemic stroke from cardiac emboli
- haemorrhagic stroke
- cerebral abscess (see Case 39)
- empyema
- venous sinus thrombosis (see Case 17).

The frequency of neurological complications in IE is in the region of 20–40% overall, of which ischaemic stroke is the most common, but the incidence varies with the infecting organism. Most neurological complications are caused by embolization, and primary infection of the CNS without prior evidence of stroke is uncommon. Unsurprisingly, systemic embolic complications are more common

Table 47.1 Modified Duke criteria for the diagnosis of infective endocarditis*

Definite infective endocarditis
Pathological criteria
Microorganisms demonstrated by culture or histological examination of a vegetation, a vegetation that has embolized, or an intracardiac abscess specimen, *or*
Pathological lesions: vegetation or intracardiac abscess confirmed by histological examination showing active endocarditis
Clinical criteria
Two major criteria, *or*
One major criterion and three minor criteria, *or*
Five minor criteria
Possible infective endocarditis
One major criterion and one minor criterion, *or*
Three minor criteria
Rejected
Firm alternative diagnosis explaining evidence of infective endocarditis, *or*
Resolution of IE syndrome with antibiotic therapy for ≤4 days, *or*
No pathological evidence of IE at surgery or autopsy, with antibiotic therapy for ≤4 days, *or*
Does not meet criteria for possible infective endocarditis as above

*Modifications to the original criteria are shown in bold type.

with left-sided cardiac involvement. Embolism from the right heart (which is more frequently involved in intravenous drug abusers than in other patients) is associated with PFO or pulmonary arteriovenous malformations. Meningitis and cerebritis follow embolization to the meninges, whereas embolization to the brain can cause micro- and macroabscesses. Macroabscesses are rare (less than 1% of neurological complications) and may occur within an area of infarction. Microabscesses are more common and may cause encephalopathy or psychosis. Embolization to the spinal meninges may cause a discitis, and embolization to the peripheral nerves may cause an ischaemic neuropathy in which persistent deep burning pain is the most common manifestation.

Around a fifth of patients with IE have an **ischaemic stroke** as a result of embolism from valvular vegetations, and the risk is thought to be higher with more virulent organisms. Infarction usually involves the cortex (and the vast majority affect the MCA territory) consistent with an embolic aetiology. Cerebrovascular symptoms are the presenting feature in around 20% of those with ischaemic stroke, but stroke usually occurs in patients who are already hospitalized but in whom infection is not controlled. Haemorrhagic transformation of infarction is fairly common (18–42%). Cerebral emboli are probably no more common than emboli to other

Table 47.2 Major and minor clinical criteria used in the modified Duke criteria

Major criteria
Blood culture positive for infective endocarditis
Typical microorganisms consistent with infective endocarditis from two separate blood cultures: Viridans streptococci, *Streptococcus bovis*, HACEK group[†], *Staphylococcus aureus*, or community-acquired enterococci in the absence of a primary focus, *or*
Microorganisms consistent with infective endocarditis from persistently positive blood cultures defined as follows: at least two positive cultures of blood samples drawn >12 hours apart, or all of three or a majority of more than four separate cultures of blood (with the first and last samples drawn at least 1 hour apart)
Single positive blood culture for *Coxiella burnetii* or anti-phase 1 IgG antibody titre >1:800
Evidence of endocardial involvement
Echocardiogram positive for infective endocarditis **(TOE recommended for patients with prosthetic valves, rated at least 'possible infective endocarditis' by clinical criteria, or complicated infective endocarditis (paravalvular abscess); TOE as first test in other patients)** defined as follows: oscillating intracardiac mass on valve or supporting structures, in the path of regurgitant jets, or on implanted material in the absence of an alternative anatomical explanation; or abscess; or new partial dehiscence of prosthetic valve; new valvular regurgitation (worsening or changing or pre-existing murmur not sufficient)

Minor criteria
Predisposition, predisposing heart condition, or injecting drug user
Fever, temperature >38°C
Vascular phenomena: major arterial emboli, septic pulmonary infarcts, mycotic aneurysm, intracranial haemorrhage, conjunctival haemorrhages, and Janeway's lesions
Immunological phenomena: glomerulonephritis, Osler's nodes, Roth's spots, and rheumatoid factor
Microbiological evidence: positive blood culture but does not meet a major criterion as noted above[‡] or serological evidence of active infection with organism consistent with infective endocarditis
Echocardiographic minor criteria eliminated

TOE, transoesophageal echocardiography; TTE, transthoracic echocardiography.
*Modifications to the original criteria are shown in bold type.
[†]HACEK group: *Haemophilus parainfluenzae*, *Haemophilus aphrophilus*, *Haemophilus paraphrophilus*, *Haemophilus influenzae*, *Actinobacillus actinomycetemcomitans*, *Cardiobacterium hominis*, *Eikenella corrodens*, *Kingella kingae*, and *Kingella kingae denitrificans*.
[‡]Excludes single positive cultures for coagulase-negative staphylococci and organisms that do not cause endocarditis.

organs, but they are more frequently reported as they are usually symptomatic and associated with increased morbidity and mortality. Occasionally, emboli to the anterior spinal artery may cause paraplegia.

IE is complicated by **intracerebral haemorrhage** in around 5% of cases. More than 80% of patients with ICH from septic emboli have a history of heart disease or intravenous drug abuse or prodromal symptoms suggestive of cerebral ischaemia.

Cerebral haemorrhage in IE is most commonly caused by **pyogenic necrosis** of the arterial wall early on in the disease, usually with virulent organisms such as *Staphylococcus aureus* and before effective treatment with antibiotics. Bleeding from ruptured mycotic aneurysms is less common, but may occur later during antimicrobial therapy or with less virulent bacteria such as *Streptococcus viridans* or *Staphylococcus epidermidis*.

Mycotic aneurysms most often affect the distal branches of the MCA. They tend to resolve with time and thus angiography to detect aneurysms with a view to surgery is generally not warranted, although some argue that it should be performed in those with haemorrhagic stroke or in whom long-term anticoagulation is being considered.

Given that fever, cardiac murmur, and abnormal echocardiography are not always present in endocarditis, the diagnosis should always be considered in any patient with otherwise unexplained ischaemic or haemorrhagic stroke, particularly if there are elevated inflammatory markers, anaemia, persistent neutrophil leucocytosis, haematuria, or disturbed liver function.

3. What further investigations would you request?

Other investigations that should be requested in this patient include:

◆ blood cultures—at least three sets taken at least 1 hour apart, ideally from different sites prior to starting antibiotics

◆ echocardiography (transthoracic and transoesophageal).

Echocardiography is mandatory to identify valvular vegetations and to assess cardiac function. Trans-thoracic echocardiography may be negative, particularly with left-sided lesions, and transoesophageal echocardiography is nearly always required.

4. How would you manage this condition?

Management of IE includes:

◆ prompt initiation of appropriate antibiotic therapy

◆ liaison with microbiologist, cardiologist and cardiothoracic surgeon

◆ consideration of cardiac surgery.

In most cases anticoagulation should not be given.

Prompt treatment with appropriate antibiotics is of paramount importance in the management of IE since this reduces the risk of complications. Independent studies have confirmed that the rate of embolic events drops dramatically during or after the first 2–3 weeks of successful antibiotic therapy. In a study published in 1991, the embolic rate dropped from 13 to less than 1.2 embolic events per 1000 patient-days during that time, and a more recent study confirmed the reduced frequency of embolization after 2 weeks of therapy and emphasized the increased risk of embolization with increasing vegetation size during therapy, mitral valve involvement, and staphylococcal causes. The prediction of risk of embolization for an individual patients remains difficult.

Identification of the causative organism is required in guiding appropriate treatment, and multiple sets of blood cultures should be taken. *Staphylococcus aureus* is the most likely causative organism in a patient who is known to use intravenous drugs. Serological tests should be taken for *Coxiella* and *Chlamydia* in patients with negative blood cultures in whom the suspicion of endocarditis remains high.

Correct management of endocarditis requires close liaison between physicians, cardiologists, microbiologists, and cardiothoracic surgeons, the last of whom should be notified even in the case of apparently stable patients as rapid deterioration may occur. Early institution of the correct antibiotic regime should be guided by microbiology advice. The indications for surgery are disputed, but valvular deterioration, infection with resistant or virulent organisms, or evidence of embolization have all been proposed. The presence of vegetations has not been consistently shown to be related to embolization, although this is used as a criterion for surgery by some. The timing of surgery in patients with stroke is also controversial, since the risks of early surgery in the presence of cerebral oedema have to be weighed against the risks of valvular deterioration or further embolization if surgery is delayed.

Early institution of the correct antibiotic therapy is the most effective way to prevent thromboembolism, the risks of which are highest in the first 24–48 hours after diagnosis. **Anticoagulation should not be given to patients with native valve or bioprosthetic valve endocarditis** because of the risk of ICH from mycotic aneurysms and arteritis and the reduction in embolism risk with antibiotic therapy. The correct management of patients with mechanical valves who are on long-term anticoagulation at the time they develop IE is unclear. Some advocate withholding anticoagulation in all such patients because it has not been shown to be associated with a reduction in the rate of systemic embolization and the risk of haemorrhagic complications with such therapy has been shown to be in the region of 40% in some studies. Others continue anticoagulation unless embolic stroke or haemorrhage occur. The length of time for which anticoagulation should be withheld is also unclear, but consultation with the cardiologists regarding the risk of embolization according to valve type may be of some help. Some authors have stated that large ischaemic stroke, haemorrhage on CT, presence of mycotic aneurysms, uncontrolled infection, and infection with *Staphylococcus aureus* are all contraindications to anticoagulants in mechanical valve endocarditis. There is no evidence for any benefit of antiplatelet therapy in ischaemic stroke secondary to IE, although animal studies suggest that such therapy may reduce vegetation size and systemic embolization.

This patient was admitted from the TIA clinic and was found to have an aortic root abscess due to an infection with a coagulase-negative staphylococcus (Fig. 47.1). She deteriorated despite antibiotics and died 2 days later. Endocarditis should always be considered in patients with cerebral ischaemia where there is evidence of infection, malaise, or new cardiac murmurs. As in this case, the symptoms may be mild and non-specific despite severe illness, especially in older patients.

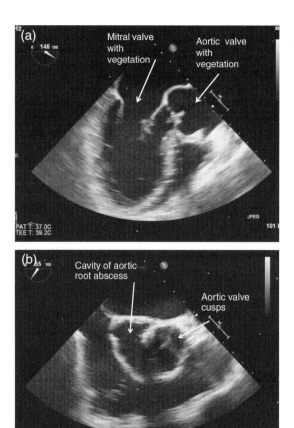

Fig. 47.1 Patient's echocardiogram. This shows vegetations on the aortic and mitral valves as indicated by the arrows. Panel (b) also shows the aortic root abscess.

Further reading

Delahaye F, Célard M, Roth O, de Gevigney G (2004). Indications and optimal timing for surgery in infective endocarditis. *Heart*; **90**: 618–20.

Derex L, Bonnefoy E, Delahaye F (2010). Impact of stroke on therapeutic decision making in infective endocarditis. *J Neurol*; **257**: 315–21.

European Society of Cardiology Guidelines: http://www.escardio.org/guidelines-surveys/esc-guidelines/Pages/infective-endocarditis.aspx.

Mugge A, Daniel WG, Frank G, Lichtlen PR (1989). Echocardiography in infective endocarditis: reassessment of prognostic implications of vegetation size determined by the transthoracic and the transesophageal approach. *J Am Coll Cardiol*; **14**: 631–8.

Sexton DJ, Spelman D (2003). Current best practices and guidelines. Assessment and management of complications in infective endocarditis. *Cardiol Clin*; **21**: 273–82, vii–viii.

Singhal AB, Topcuoglu MA, Buonanno FS (2002). Acute ischemic stroke patterns in infective and nonbacterial thrombotic endocarditis: a diffusion-weighted magnetic resonance imaging study. *Stroke*; **33**: 1267–73.

Vilacosta I, Graupner C, San Roman JA, *et al.* (2002). Risk of embolization after institution of antibiotic therapy for infective endocarditis. *J Am Coll Cardiol*; **39**: 1489–95.

Case 48

A 35-year-old man was decorating his living room. After lifting a pot of paint, he became aware of a tingling sensation in his right arm. When he resumed painting, he had difficulty handling the brush. His wife noticed that he had a facial weakness and that his speech was slurred. The symptoms resolved 2 days later. The patient had a long history of migraine with visual aura, but was otherwise healthy and was not on any medication. He had never smoked and only rarely drank alcohol. He had returned from a trekking holiday in Nepal a week earlier. MRI brain with DWI showed a small cortical infarct in the left MCA territory.

Questions

1. How would you investigate this patient further?
2. Do you think the history of migraine with aura is of any relevance?
3. What are the treatment options in this patient?

Answers

1. How would you investigate this patient further?

This patient has had a stroke, possibly in association with a Valsalva manoeuvre. Given the circumstances in which this stroke occurred, there are two main differential diagnoses. First, the lifting and associated Valsalva manoeuvre may have caused a carotid dissection with either vessel occlusion or thrombus formation and embolization. Secondly, the Valsalva manoeuvre associated with lifting a heavy object may have caused a paradoxical embolus through a right-to-left shunt such as a PFO. As the patient had been on a long-haul flight just a week earlier, he may have developed a deep vein thrombosis from which the embolus could have formed. The patient should have imaging of his cervical vessels with either MRA or CTA to look for a carotid dissection. He should also have an echocardiogram to look for potential cardioembolic sources. This should be done with bubble contrast (agitated saline) to look for a PFO as the most common pathway for a paradoxical embolus. Usually a TTE is done first, followed by a transoesophageal echocardiogram (TOE) if the TTE has not shown a PFO or other embolic source. The advantage of the TOE is that it provides a better view of the left atrium. However, a small right-to-left shunt through a PFO may only be visible while the patient is doing a Valsalva manoeuvre. This can be difficult with a TOE probe in place, and a TTE may be preferable in slim patients. An alternative way of looking for a right-to-left shunt is with transcranial Doppler: agitated saline is injected, and the transcranial Doppler probe, which is placed over the MCA, will show high-intensity transient signals (HITS), when an air bubble from the agitated saline passes. The number of HITS, and whether they occur at rest or only with Valsalva, provides some information about the size of the shunt. However, transcranial Doppler does not provide any structural information about the shunt. Nevertheless, a potential advantage is that it also shows up the presence of non-cardiac shunts (e.g. pulmonary shunts), which will be missed on echocardiography.

If a PFO is detected, the next step should be to try and locate the source of the thrombus. However, this may be difficult or too invasive in proximal thrombosis (e.g. the pelvic veins). Venous Doppler of the legs is often normal. Nevertheless, young patients with a suspected or proven thrombosis should be investigated for a thrombophilic tendency, in particular in the absence of obvious risk factors or if there is a history of previous thromboembolic events. In our patient, TTE showed a large PFO with an atrial septal aneurysm (ASA). A venous Doppler scan of the legs was normal, as was thrombophilia screening.

2. Do you think the history of migraine with aura is of any relevance?

In our patient, the combination of having a PFO and migraine with aura may be due to more than chance. Several studies have proposed that the prevalence of PFOs is higher in people with migraine with aura than in people without migraine. There have also been several reports that attacks of migraine with aura decreased in frequency or stopped if a patient's PFO was closed. A possible explanation for the somewhat surprising association between migraine with aura and a PFO is that the PFO allows the passage of vasoactive substances, which would normally be metabolized in the lungs, into the arterial circulation where they can then cause migraine. However, a randomized trial of PFO closure in patients with migraine with aura failed to show any significant benefit of intervention. In addition, more recent larger studies have failed to show an association between migraine and PFO ovale, and the current view is that such a relationship does not exist.

Migraine with aura *per se* also is a risk factor for stroke (see Case 7). This relative increase in risk conferred by migraine is particularly obvious in women, especially if they are under the age of 45 years, smoke, and are on the oral contraceptive pill. The mechanism by which migraine with aura increases the risk of ischaemic vascular events is uncertain.

3. What are the treatment options in this patient?

Treatment should be directed at preventing further events. In our patient, the main question is whether his stroke is due to the PFO, and if so, what the risk of recurrence is.

A PFO occurs in about 25% of the general population. Therefore its presence in someone who has had a stroke may be purely coincidental. However, the prevalence of a PFO is higher in patients with cryptogenic stroke than in controls without stroke. This higher prevalence is particularly marked in patients younger than 55 years, but it persists in older patients. The prevalence of a PFO combined with an ASA is particularly high in stroke patients compared with controls, suggesting that this may confer a higher stroke risk. However, while these associations point towards an association of PFO and stroke, they give no information about the risk of recurrent stroke. Studies give a wide range of recurrent event rates. A recent meta-analysis gave a pooled risk of 1.6 strokes per 100 patient years of follow-up. It showed that, overall, the risk of recurrence in patients with cryptogenic stroke and a PFO is not higher than in cryptogenic stroke patients without a PFO.

These data suggest that no particular treatment is required for a PFO. However, in some patients, the association between their stroke and a PFO appears to be strong, and they may be at a higher risk of further events. Such a strong association is suggested by a Valsalva manoeuvre at the time of the event and by a prothrombotic state. Both of these were present in our patient, and he also had an ASA. Therefore more specific treatment of his PFO seemed justified.

Treatment options include medical treatment with either aspirin or anticoagulation, and interventional treatment with either surgical or endovascular PFO closure. For medical treatment, there is insufficient evidence to determine if either aspirin or anticoagulation is superior, but the risk of minor haemorrhage is increased with anticoagulation. Nevertheless, any of the potential mechanisms by which a PFO could cause a stroke (i.e. a paradoxical embolus, embolization of thrombus originating at the PFO, or thrombus formation caused by intermittent arrhythmias) would usually be an indication for anticoagulation. Surgical closure of a PFO requires a thoracotomy with all its associated risks, and this procedure is now rarely performed. The current preferred method of closing a PFO is with an umbrella device which can be placed across the inter-atrial septum with an endovascular approach. This is a low-risk procedure, but complications in the form of device breakage or embolization, thrombus formation on the device, or bacterial endocarditis may still occur.

Our patient underwent endovascular closure of his PFO, and he also continues to take aspirin. He has had no further events, and he has not noticed any change in the character or frequency of his migraine. Overall too little is still known about whether PFO closure reduces the risk of recurrent stroke compared with medical treatment, and which medical treatment might be best. Trials are ongoing. Until more data are available, the recommendation has to be to manage patients with cryptogenic stroke and PFO conservatively. If their history is strongly suggestive of a paradoxical embolus and if they appear to be at high risk of further events or have multiple events, PFO closure should be considered or they should be enrolled in one of the trials.

Further reading

Almekhlafi MA, Wilton SB, Rabi DM, *et al.* (2009). Recurrent cerebral ischemia in medically treated patent foramen ovale: a meta-analysis. *Neurology*; **73**; 89–97.

Garg P, Servoss SJ, Wu JC, *et al.* (2010). Lack of association between migraine headache and patent foramen ovale: results of a case–control study. *Circulation*; **121**: 1406–12.

Overell JR, Bone I, Lees K (2000). Interatrial septal abnormalities and stroke: a meta-analysis of case–control studies. *Neurology*; **55**: 1172–9.

Schürks M, Rist PM, Biga ME, *et al.* (2009). Migraine and cardiovascular disease: systematic review and meta-analysis. *BMJ*; **339**: b3914.

Case 49

An 80-year-old woman was admitted with slurred speech and collapse after having been found slumped to the left in a chair by a carer. She lived alone, with care three times daily, and was usually mobile with a Zimmer frame. Although the carer thought that her speech had been normal prior to the collapse, her daughter thought that it had been slightly slurred for the previous weeks and had suddenly become worse on the day of admission. The patient's mobility had also been declining over the preceding months and she had fallen several times. She had also developed some urinary incontinence. There was a past medical history of type 2 diabetes and hypertension, and she had known left ventricular hypertrophy.

On examination, she was apyrexial, pulse was 70bpm regular, and blood pressure was 170/90mmHg. Heart sounds were normal, but respiratory examination showed reduced air entry and crepitations at the right base. Nervous system examination showed severe dysarthria (pseudobulbar in character) such that her speech was unintelligible, increased tone throughout the limbs, reduced proximal limb power, brisk symmetrical reflexes, and extensor plantars. Review by speech and language therapy showed a spastic palate with delayed swallow, and she was advised thickened fluids and soft diet.

Investigations showed the following:

◆ CRP 103, WCC 13.6

◆ CXR showed evidence of right-sided consolidation

◆ CT and MRI brain scans are shown in Fig. 49.1

Questions

1. What do the scans in Fig. 49.1 show? Does this help diagnostically? What are the neuropathological substrates of these changes?

2. Give a differential diagnosis for the neurological features in this case. What is the most likely diagnosis? What is the most likely cause of the elevated CRP and CXR changes?

3. How would you manage this condition and what is the prognosis?

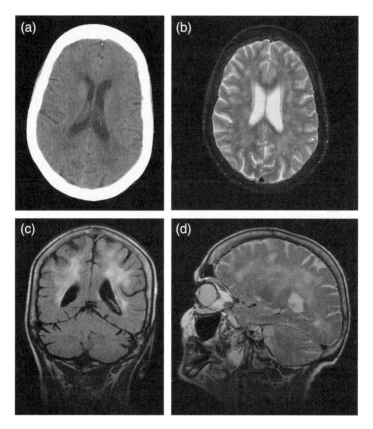

Fig. 49.1 CT brain (a), axial T2-weighted MRI (b), coronal FLAIR image (c) and sagittal T2-weighted MRI (d).

Answers

1. What do the scans in Fig. 49.1 show? Does this help diagnostically? What are the neuropathological substrates of these changes?

The CT and MRI scans show extensive confluent white matter abnormalities. The differential diagnosis for such appearances depends on the age of the patient and the clinical picture. In general, a much wider differential diagnosis must be considered in younger patients. The extensive white matter changes on the brain imaging are not specific, and while they may provide an explanation for this patient's symptoms, other differential diagnoses should also be considered (see also Question 2).

In elderly patients, the most common aetiology of diffuse radiological white matter abnormality is small vessel ischaemic change or leukoaraiosis. In younger patients, storage diseases and acute demyelinating encephalomyelitis (ADEM) should be considered, but the clinical presentation would be different to the current case. Other more uncommon causes of diffuse white matter changes, which have been found in post-mortem series, include disseminated white matter metastases, lymphoma, and obstructive hydrocephalus.

The term 'leukoaraiosis' is derived from the Greek stem *leuko-*, meaning white and referring to the white matter, and the adjective *araios* meaning rarefied. Leukoaraiosis is defined as diffuse confluent white matter abnormality (low density on CT, high signal on T2-weighted or FLAIR MRI), often with irregular margins. As a purely radiological concept, the term could equally be applied to the leukodystrophies, as well as some metabolic and inflammatory disorders. The vascular and degenerative forms of leukoaraiosis are most common (see Table 49.1).

The white matter of the cerebral hemispheres is largely supplied by long narrow penetrating arteries and arterioles that arise from branches of the major cerebral arteries on the pial surface of the brain. In regions of leukoaraiosis, alterations in the structure of these vessels are an invariable feature. The major pathological findings in leukoaraiosis are myelin pallor, enlargement of perivascular spaces, gliosis, and axonal loss. Fazekas and colleagues demonstrated that in asymptomatic older adults pathological heterogeneity diminishes as lesion severity increases from small punctate hyperintensities to early confluent and then confluent lesions, which almost always have an ischaemic appearance with myelin loss, gliosis, and micro-infarction. In contrast, periventricular 'caps' and a smooth halo (or 'band') around the lateral ventricles have a non-ischaemic appearance with subependymal gliosis and discontinuity of the ependymal lining.

Leukoaraiosis is associated with age, hypertension, history of stroke (particularly small vessel disease, i.e. lacunar stroke), and dementia. Leukoaraiosis is common in vascular dementia, but is also seen in up to 30% of those with 'pure' AD. Given its association with AD and predilection for small arteries, CAA might seem the most obvious cause of leukoaraiosis in AD (see Case 6). However, it appears that leukoaraiosis co-localizes with, and correlates with, the severity of non-amyloid

Table 49.1 Vascular causes of leukoaraiosis in older adults

Diagnostic group	Common clinical associations	Diagnosis	Main pathological abnormality of small vessels	Radiological features
Ischaemic leukoaraiosis	Lacunar stroke/TIA Established risk factors: age and hypertension Emerging risk factors: homocysteine	History of lacunar stroke/TIA	Arteriosclerosis ('simple' small vessel disease) Lipohyalinosis ('complex' small vessel disease)	Lacunar infarcts
Sporadic CAA (see Case 6)	Lobar haemorrhage Ischaemic stroke Cognitive impairment	Boston Criteria (in brief): >55 years Multiple cortical or juxtacortical bleeds No other cause of haemorrhage	Amyloid deposits in proximal portions of penetrating arteries/arterioles (consisting mostly of $A\beta_{1-40}$)	Cortical/ juxtacortical micro-haemorrhages Superficial SAH
CADASIL (see Case 28)	Lacunar stroke/TIA Migraine Depressive symptoms Cognitive impairment Familial history of the above	Notch 3 genetic testing Skin biopsy	Granular osmiophilic material and loss of smooth muscle cells in the media of small arteries	Anterior temporal pole hyperintensity on T2 MRI Lacunar infarcts and micro-haemorrhages

arteriosclerosis. Leukoaraiosis is also increasingly recognized as a feature of sporadic CAA (see Case 6) without AD. Leukoaraiosis is found in some of the genetic amyloid angiopathies (e.g. familial British dementia), suggesting that amyloid angiopathy alone is sufficient to cause this imaging appearance.

Leukoaraiosis and small vessel disease

Pathological studies suggest that leukoaraiosis is one manifestation of cerebral small vessel disease. This is supported by strong pathological and clinical associations with the other major manifestation of small vessel disease: lacunar stroke. However, although leukoaraiosis and lacunar infarcts are often found together, in individual patients one type of imaging appearance may predominate: leukoaraiosis or isolated lacunar infarcts (multiple lacunar lesions but no leukoaraiosis on imaging). Essentially this is the modern-day imaging analogue of the distinction between diffuse white matter pathology and a state of multiple discrete lacunar infarcts described by Pierre Marie in 1901 and christened *état lacunaire*. These two imaging types have recently been shown to differ in their risk factor profile; age and hypertension are most strongly associated with ischaemic leukoaraiosis while hypercholesterolaemia, diabetes mellitus, and myocardial infarction are more associated with isolated lacunar infarction. These findings suggest some differences in pathogenesis, with leukoaraiosis perhaps reflecting a non-atheromatous pathology of smaller-calibre vessels than those implicated in lacunar infarcts.

2. Give a differential diagnosis for the neurological features in this case. What is the most likely diagnosis? What is the most likely cause of the elevated CRP and CXR changes?

The differential diagnosis in this patient includes:

◆ acute cerebrovascular event

◆ severe subcortical white matter disease

◆ motor neuron disease

◆ myasthenia gravis.

The most likely diagnosis is severe **subcortical white matter disease** causing dysarthria, reduced mobility, and incontinence, with decompensation secondary to aspiration and **chest sepsis** (causing the CXR changes and elevated inflammatory markers).

The clinical features of this case illustrate the relatively common scenario of an elderly patient with significant comorbidity presenting with collapse and slumping to one side. In such cases, the working diagnosis in the emergency room is almost always one of stroke. In this patient, there were underlying vascular risk factors and a history of sudden onset, or at least sudden worsening of dysarthria. There were no other focal neurological signs but there was increased tone and upgoing plantars, indicating damage to the descending motor pathways. The assumption was of a **brainstem ischaemic event**. However, the history of preceding slurring of speech together with progressive decline in mobility and urinary incontinence suggest that this patient's symptoms are not all acute. The CT and MRI findings of extensive and confluent white matter changes in association with dysarthria, gait disturbance, and cognitive decline correspond to the classical descriptions of Binswanger's disease.

In 1894, in a paper on the differential diagnosis of general paralysis of the insane, Otto Binswanger linked marked atrophy of the cerebral white matter and arteriosclerosis to a syndrome of progressive decline of mental functions with depression and personality change, diminished power in the legs, and tremor. Some of the classical features of the early descriptions of 'Binswanger's disease', including dementia, pseudobulbar palsy, and gait disturbance are now rare, and it seems likely that many of the original Binswanger patients had neurosyphilis rather than age-related small vessel disease. However, as the current case illustrates, the clinical features of Binswanger's disease may still occur. Nevertheless, today Binswanger's disease is a somewhat controversial entity. Many of the features of classical Binswanger's disease occur in patients with vascular cognitive impairment, but it should be noted that not all older patients with severe white matter disease have cognitive impairment; marked physical disability may occur in the presence of well-preserved cognition.

Motor neuron disease should always be considered in patients presenting with dysarthria (see Case 27). In this patient, there were no lower motor neuron signs and the tongue was not wasted. However, the diagnosis cannot be excluded on the basis of the clinical findings at this point. Similarly, **myasthenia gravis** is an important cause of dysarthria and weakness but it does not explain the spastic nature of the dysarthria or the limb findings in this case. The differential diagnosis of dysarthria is discussed in Case 27.

Rapid cognitive decline and deteriorating gait over weeks to a few months should also prompt consideration of other causes such as normal pressure hydrocephalus, malignancy, or inflammatory brain disorders.

3. How would you manage this condition and what is the prognosis?

Management of severe leukoaraiosis is supportive. The prognosis of severe leukoaraiosis is poor.

Patients with severe leukoaraiosis are at increased risk of cognitive decline, poor mobility, falls, incontinence, and dependency. Both lacunes and confluent white matter changes are independently associated with cognitive changes, particularly executive deficits and slowing of processing speed. Cognitive function should therefore be assessed with tests sensitive to frontal and executive function (see Case 8). There has been a continuing debate on whether periventricular or deep leukoaraiosis is more damaging to cognition. In the Rotterdam Scan Study, periventricular leukoaraiosis (and infarcts), but not subcortical white matter lesions, were correlated with a decline in processing speed. Periventricular lesions affect cholinergic projections, as assessed by positron emission tomography. The LADIS study found that lacunar infarcts in the thalamus are especially likely to damage cognition in several domains, whereas those in the putamen and pallidum may have an effect on memory. Lacunes in the internal capsule, lobar white matter, and caudate had no detectable cognitive consequences.

Up to 80% of patients with leukoaraiosis have a gait disorder which is associated with an increased risk of falls. Falls and balance disturbances are associated primarily with frontal deep and periventricular leukoaraiosis that is thought to cause interruption of frontal lobe circuits. Walking difficulties may be the main presenting feature of leukoaraiosis, particularly when exacerbated by intercurrent illness (as in the current case), and may be a common manifestation of leukoaraiosis in patients who present 'off legs' to acute medical services.

Leukoaraiosis progresses with time. In the Rotterdam Scan Study of 668 people with a mean age of 71 years at their first scan, 39% showed visible progression of leukoaraiosis at 3 years (32% subcortical, 27% periventricular) along with a 14% incidence of silent infarcts and a 2% incidence of symptomatic infarcts. In the PROGRESS trial, no leukoaraiosis at study entry was associated with a 4% risk of dementia or severe cognitive decline after 4 years of follow-up versus a 30% risk in those with severe leukoaraiosis at entry. The LADIS study has also now reported 2.4-year follow-up data for its observational cohort of 633 74-year-olds and found a very similar transition rate of 29.5% to death or disability in activities of daily living for those with severe leukoaraiosis at entry versus 10% in those with only mild changes. Baseline severity of leukoaraiosis, age, blood pressure, current smoking, and the presence of lacunar infarcts predict progression. Progression of periventricular lesions results in decline in MMSE score, whereas subcortical leukoaraiosis has fewer cognitive effects.

In several prospective studies, leukoaraiosis has been associated with an increased risk of ischaemic stroke, cerebral haemorrhage, vascular death, and all-cause mortality. Increased mortality occurs not just through stroke and vascular death but also via an increased risk of pneumonia and falls, as illustrated in the current case.

Further reading

Baezner H, Blahak C, Poggesi A, *et al.* (2008). Association of gait and balance disorders with age-related white matter changes: the LADIS study. *Neurology*; **70**: 935–42.

Benisty S, Gouw AA, Porcher R, *et al.* (2009). Location of lacunar infarcts correlates with cognition in a sample of non-disabled subjects with age-related white-matter changes: the LADIS study. *J Neurol Neurosurg Psychiatry*; **80**: 478–83.

Blahak C, Baezner H, Pantoni L, *et al.* (2009). Deep frontal and periventricular age related white matter changes but not basal ganglia and infratentorial hyperintensities are associated with falls: cross sectional results from the LADIS study. *J Neurol Neurosurg Psychiatry*; **80**: 608–13.

Bohnen NI, Muller MLTM, Kuwabara H, Constantine GM, Studenski SA (2009). Age-associated leukoaraiosis and cortical cholinergic deafferentation. *Neurology*; **72**: 1411–16.

Dufouil C, Godin O, Chalmers J, *et al.* (2009). Severe cerebral white matter hyperintensities predict severe cognitive decline in patients with cerebrovascular disease history. *Stroke*; **40**: 2219–21.

Inzitari D, Simoni M, Pracucci G, *et al.* (2007). Risk of rapid global functional decline in elderly patients with severe cerebral age-related white matter changes: the LADIS study. *Arch Intern Med*; **167**: 81–8.

Inzitari D, Pracucci G, Poggesi A, *et al.* (2009). Changes in white matter as determinant of global functional decline in older independent outpatients: three year follow-up of LADIS (Leukoaraiosis and Disability) study cohort. *BMJ*; **339**: b2477.

Jokinen H, Kalska H, Ylikoski R, *et al.* (2009) MRI-defined subcortical ischemic vascular disease: baseline clinical and neuropsychological findings. The LADIS study. *Cerebrovasc Dis*; **27**: 336–44.

Jokinen H, Kalska H, Ylikoski R, *et al.* (2009). Longitudinal cognitive decline in subcortical ischemic vascular disease: the LADIS study. *Cerebrovasc Dis*; **27**: 384–91.

Ropele S, Seewann A, Gouw AA, *et al.* (2009). Quantitation of brain tissue changes associated with white matter hyperintensities by diffusion-weighted and magnetization transfer imaging:the LADIS (Leukoaraiosis and Disability in the Elderly) study. *J Magn Reson Imaging*; **29**: 268–74.

van der Flier WM, van Straaten EC, Barkhof F, *et al.* (2005). Small vessel disease and general cognitive function in nondisabled elderly: the LADIS study. *Stroke*; **36**: 2116–20.

van Dijk EJ, Prins ND, Vrooman HA, Hofman A, Koudstaal PJ, Breteler MMB (2008). Progression of cerebral small-vessel disease in relation to risk factors and cognitive consequences: Rotterdam Scan Study. *Stroke*; **39**: 2712–19.

Verdelho A, Madureira S, Moleiro C, *et al.* (2010). White matter changes and diabetes predict cognitive decline in the elderly: the LADIS study. *Neurology*; **75**: 160–7.

Case 50

An 87-year-old retired forklift truck driver was admitted with confusion and being 'off legs'. His daughters reported that they had found he was confused during a telephone call and on going to investigate had found him sitting on a stool unable to get up. There was a past history of hypertension and peripheral vascular disease. He was taking aspirin and antihypertensive medication.

On examination, he was apyrexial with GCS 14/15 (losing a point for confused speech) and normal pulse and blood pressure. There was mild left flank tenderness but no neck stiffness and no focal neurological signs. He scored 8/10 on the abbreviated mental test, losing points for orientation. He was reviewed by the surgical team because of his flank pain, and a CT abdomen was done which also showed lymphadenopathy and splenomegaly (Fig. 50.1). The following morning he was found to be extremely drowsy, although he was rousable and responded appropriately to simple questions and commands. His blood sugar was normal but he was pyrexial with a temperature of 38.3°C. The rest of the neurological examination did not reveal any abnormalities. Given the sudden deterioration in level of consciousness, a CT brain was done (Fig. 50.2).

Over the next 2 days the patient's level of consciousness gradually deteriorated further, until on day 3 his GCS was 3/15. The neurological examination at that point revealed bilateral extensor plantar responses, small but reactive pupils, and increased tone in the right arm and leg. MRI brain was performed (Fig. 50.3).

Further investigations showed the following:

- Hb 10.9; WCC 1.9 (0.69 neutrophils); platelets 171; PT 14.6; activated partial thromboplastin time (APPT) 45.9
- Na 131; K 4.7; urea 9.9; Cr 116; CRP 24; Ca 2.18
- LFT normal; LDH 187
- Blood cultures negative
- Urine dipstick negative
- CXR: mild cardiomegaly, some left lower lobe consolidation

Questions

1. What is the abnormality on the CT brain?
2. What does the MRI brain show?
3. What is the cause of this man's gradual descent into coma?
4. Is there a unifying diagnosis that explains the findings on the CT abdomen, the full blood count, and the MRI brain?

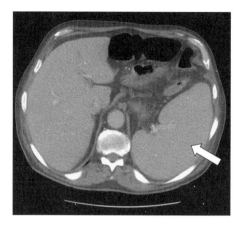

Fig. 50.1 The CT abdomen showing splenomegaly (arrow).

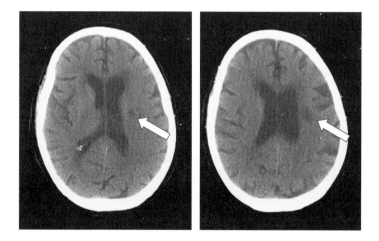

Fig. 50.2 CT brain.

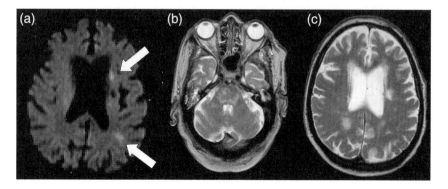

Fig. 50.3 MRI brain: DWI (a) and axial T2-weighted images ((b) and (c)).

Answers

1. What is the abnormality on the CT brain?

The CT brain scan shows a lacunar infarct (arrow) and widespread signal change in the subcortical white matter, most likely due to cerebral small vessel disease.

2. What does the MRI brain show?

The MRI brain scan shows multiple ischaemic lesions. These are located in the mid-brain, the right thalamus, and the subcortical white matter of both hemispheres. Some of the lesions, in particular the left hemispheric subcortical lesions, appear acute on DWI (Fig. 50.3 (a), arrows). There are also chronic ischaemic changes, and there is diffuse signal change in the subcortical white matter and the brainstem which is suggestive of small vessel disease.

The brain imaging findings illustrate how insensitive CT brain may be in acute stroke. The CT findings were not particularly remarkable, particularly for an elderly patient, and yet the MRI showed extensive abnormalities prompting a search for an underlying cause that would explain his multiple acute infarctions (see also Case 4).

3. What is the cause of this man's gradual descent into coma?

This man's gradual descent into coma is most likely related to the occurrence of multiple episodes of acute cerebral infarction. Specifically, he has bilateral ischaemic lesions in the brainstem, which extend into the pons, and he also has a thalamic infarct. Both these locations can be associated with decreased level of consciousness. In addition to the ischaemic lesions, there may also be an associated encephalopathy from metabolic changes, and widespread global cerebral ischaemia including in areas not overtly infarcted. The patient died 2 weeks after presentation.

4. Is there a unifying diagnosis that explains the findings on the CT abdomen, the full blood count, and the MRI brain?

The unifying diagnosis is intravascular large B-cell lymphoma (IVBCL).

The prominent features in this patient's presentation are multiple cerebral infarcts in multiple vascular territories, which are of different ages and include multiple recent infarcts. He also has evidence of an underlying systemic disorder. Pyrexia and lymphadenopathy could point towards an inflammatory process, but his pancytopenia and splenomegaly are more suggestive of a haematological disorder.

The presence of multiple areas of infarction in different vascular territories raises the possibility of cardioembolism. **Infective endocarditis** (see Case 47) causes pyrexia, cardioembolism, and splenomegaly, but there were no signs of systemic emboli or large volume cerebral infarction caused by occlusion of large rather than purely small vessels, and IE does not explain the pancytopenia or CT abdomen findings. **Cerebral vasculitis** (see Cases 11 and 25) may cause identical radiological findings to those seen in the current case and often encephalopathy with changes in level of consciousness. However, pancytopenia would not usually be a feature in the absence of immunosuppressive therapy and the other clinical features are not consistent with this diagnosis.

IVBCL is a rare form of diffuse large B-cell lymphoma characterized by preferential intravascular growth of malignant lymphocytes in small and medium-sized vessels. The disease is aggressive and often rapidly fatal. Patients are usually elderly and frail, and men and women appear equally affected. Symptoms include general decline, fatigue, fever, and alteration in neurological function, and their non-specific nature means that many patients are only diagnosed post-mortem.

Any organ may be involved in IVBCL, including the CNS, lymphatic system, skin, spleen, and bone marrow. Typically, patients present with fever, dyspnoea, cough, and CNS signs including decreased level of consciousness, global cognitive impairment, disorientation, and focal neurological deficits such as limb weakness or speech disturbance. The patient described in the current case deteriorated extremely rapidly, such that a bone marrow or other tissue sample was not obtained. However, many of the features of this case, including the splenomegaly, fever, low haemoglobin, and neutropenia, are typical of IVBCL. Splenic venous involvement, as suggested by the findings on the CT abdomen in this patient, is typical of IVBCL.

Brain imaging findings in IVBCL are varied, and up to 50% of patients with neurological abnormalities may have normal imaging (cf. systemic lupus erythematosus). However, multiple white matter abnormalities consistent with multiple small infarcts are often seen, and these appearances may be indistinguishable from CNS vasculitis (see Fig. 50.4). MRA may also be abnormal, with narrowing of vessels and beading, which again can appear very similar to vasculitis.

Other haematological cancers may also be associated with stroke. Hyperleukocytic leukaemias are associated with hyperviscocity and may occlude small cerebral vessels leading to microinfarcts and petechial haemorrhages resulting in global neurological dysfunction (i.e. encephalopathy). In both leukaemia and lymphoma, especially acute myelogenous leukaemias, acute disseminated intravascular coagulation (DIC) may occur and lead to systemic and brain haemorrhages which may be fulminant. Bleeding usually occurs in the brain or subdural compartment, and rarely in the subarachnoid space. The diagnosis can be suspected by the clinical setting and by systemic thrombosis or haemorrhage. It can be established by examination of the peripheral blood smear, the platelet count, and tests of coagulation function.

Post-mortem findings in this case showed the presence of lymphoma cells in the small arteries which stained positive with an antibody against B lymphocytes. The pathological diagnosis was of malignant intravascular lymphoma causing multiple cerebral infarcts.

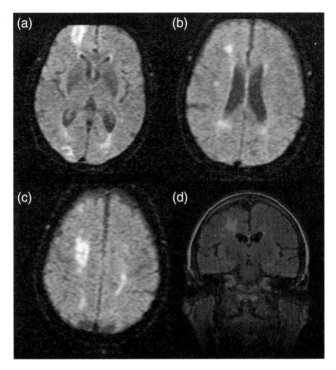

Fig. 50.4 Brain imaging from another case of IVBCL: (a)–(c) DWI showing multifocal subcortical areas of signal change within the anterior and posterior circulation, maximal in the right frontal lobe, in keeping with acute infarction; (d) coronal FLAIR image showing right frontal infarction.

Further reading

Baehring JM, Longtine J, Hochberg FH (2003). A new approach to the diagnosis and treatment of intravascular lymphoma. *J Neurooncol*; **61**: 237–48.

Ponzoni M, Ferreri AJ, Campo E, *et al.* (2007). Definition, diagnosis, and management of intravascular large B-cell lymphoma: proposals and perspectives from an international consensus meeting. *J Clin Oncol*; **25**: 3168–73.

Rogers LR (2003). Cerebrovascular complications in cancer patients. *Neurol Clin*; **21**: 167–92.

Shimada K, Kinoshita T, Naoe T, Nakamura S (2009). Presentation and management of intravascular large B-cell lymphoma. *Lancet Oncol*; **10**: 895–902.

Zuckerman D, Seliem R, Hochberg E (2006). Intravascular lymphoma: the oncologist's 'great imitator. *Oncologist*; **11**: 496–502.

Case 51

Case 51.A

A 72-year-old woman was found by her husband at 01.00 after she had fallen out of bed. She looked confused, and although she was trying to raise herself from the floor and reply to her husband's questions, she was unable to do so. When she had gone to bed at 23.30, she had been completely well. Her husband called an ambulance, and the woman arrived at the accident and emergency department at 01.45 She had a right sensory motor hemiparesis and was dysphasic. Blood pressure was 160/95mmHg, and heart rate was 92bpm regular. Her only past medical history was of hypertension and mild diabetes, for which she was taking an ACE inhibitor and metformin. She had never smoked.

Questions

1. What is the likely diagnosis? Give some differential diagnoses.

2. What investigations would you do next?

3. How would you treat this patient?

Answers

1. What is the likely diagnosis? Give some differential diagnoses.

The most likely diagnosis is that this woman has had an ischaemic stroke, most likely an infarct in the left MCA territory. These infarcts are most frequently of embolic origin, from either large vessel atheroma or a cardioembolic source. Other options include arterial dissection (see Case 24) or rare causes such as vasculitis (see Cases 11 and 15). However, these are uncommon, and are unlikely in the current setting. Although 80–85% of all strokes are ischaemic, this woman may also have had a cerebral haemorrhage. Other differential diagnoses include hypoglycaemia, a postictal state after a focal left hemispheric seizure (see Case 42), migraine (see Case 7), or encephalitis. However, for virtually all of these there should be a history of either a prodrome or previous similar events.

2. What investigations would you do next?

The main differential is between an ischaemic and a haemorrhagic cerebrovascular event. The only way to differentiate between these two is by brain imaging, either with CT or MRI. CT will clearly show any haemorrhage, and it may also show some early ischaemic changes. MRI with DWI may show the extent of any ischaemic lesions more clearly, and it will also show haemorrhage. However, currently it is less widely available acutely, and as patients have to lie still, it will also be more difficult to obtain high-quality images from a potentially poorly cooperative patient. In addition to brain imaging, blood sugar should be checked, and basic bloods (including full blood count, coagulation screen, serum electrolytes, blood glucose, CRP, liver, and renal function) sent off. An ECG to identify any cardiac arrhythmia or associated cardiac ischaemia should also be done. No other investigations are routinely required at the acute stage.

3. How would you treat this patient?

This woman has probably had an acute ischaemic stroke, and she has no obvious contraindications to thrombolysis. She was last seen well at 23.30; therefore this is the time that would count as time of symptom onset. She arrived at 01.45, i.e. 2 hours and 15 minutes after the presumed symptom onset. She still falls within the 3 hour time window for thrombolysis, and more recent studies have shown that thrombolysis is safe and of benefit for up to 4.5 hours after symptom onset although the benefit decreases with increasing time since the event. This woman should have urgent brain imaging. If this excludes a haemorrhage or other lesion, and perhaps confirms the presence of 'early infarct signs', and if there are no contraindications, thrombolysis is indicated and should be started as quickly as possible. The dose for tissue plasminogen activator (TPA) is 0.9mg/kg bodyweight, with a maximum dose of 90mg; 10% is given as a bolus and the remainder over 1 hour. The patient's heart rate, blood pressure, and neurological status should be monitored throughout; blood pressure must stay below 185/110mmHg. The patient should not be given any antiplatelet drugs or anticoagulation for 24 hours after thrombolysis, and follow-up brain imaging to assess final infarct size and possible haemorrhagic complications should be arranged for the next day or sooner if there are complications. Vascular imaging, in particular of the intracranial vessels to look for the site of vessel occlusion, is increasingly done at the acute stage in case intra-arterial intervention may be considered. Further investigations to identify the aetiology of the stroke, namely imaging of the cervical vessels to look for large artery stenosis and cardiac investigations to identify possible cardioembolism, should be done as soon as possible after the acute treatment to initiate appropriate secondary prevention therapy.

Table 51.1 shows the indications and contraindications for IV thrombolysis. The only potential contraindication in this woman is that she might have sustained a head injury when falling out of bed. However, there was no bruising or any other injury, and there were no hard objects in the vicinity, so the risk of a significant head injury was thought to be minimal.

Table 51.1 Indications and contraindications for thrombolysis according to NINDS Criteria*

Indications for thrombolysis
Diagnosis: ischaemic stroke with measurable neurological deficit
deficit should not be resolving spontaneously
deficit should not be minor and isolated
Symptom onset <3 hours (4.5 hours) before starting treatment
Patient and family understand potential risks and benefits of treatment
Contraindications for thrombolysis
Symptoms suggestive of subarachnoid haemorrhage
Head trauma or prior stroke in previous 3 months
Myocardial infarction in previous 3 months
Gastrointestinal or urinary tract haemorrhage in previous 21 days
Major surgery in previous 14 days
Arterial puncture at a non-compressible site in previous 7 days
History of previous intracranial hemorrhage
Evidence of active bleeding or acute trauma (fracture) on examination
Seizure at onset with postictal deficit (relative contraindication)
Blood pressure ≥185mmHg systolic and/or 110mmHg diastolic
Oral anticoagulation: if on anticoagulants, INR must be ≤1.5 to allow thrombolysis
Not on heparin: if on heparin in previous 48 hours, APTT must be in normal range to allow thrombolysis.
Platelet count <100 000/mm^3
Blood glucose concentration <2.7mmol/L
Multilobar infarction on CT (hypodensity >1/3 cerebral hemisphere).

*See Adams *et al.* 2007

Case 51.B

A 40-year-old man presented to the emergency department with a 90-minute history of right face, hand, and leg weakness and dysarthria. CT brain showed an area consistent with established infarction in the left caudate and lentiform nuclei. There was no past history of stroke and no vascular risk factors. He was not taking any medication.

Questions

1. Give a differential diagnosis. How are the CT changes relevant to your differential?
2. What further information is needed to guide decision making with respect to thrombolysis?

Answers

1. Give a differential diagnosis. How are the CT changes relevant to your differential?

This patient presented with a short history of a right hemiparesis, which could suggest a vascular aetiology. However, he is young and has no vascular risk factors, so he is an unusual patient to have a stroke. Other potential diagnoses include hemiplegic migraine, hypoglycaemia, Todd's palsy, and psychogenic weakness (see Case 20). These should be looked for in the history.

Given that the patient's symptoms only started 90 minutes previously, it is very unlikely that the lesion on the CT is responsible for the current symptoms, as after this time span a CT is usually still normal and it is certainly too early for an infarct to have become established. However, the lesion, if it really is due to an infarct, may indicate that the patient has had an ischaemic event previously and therefore that the current presentation is also more likely to be due to a cerebral ischaemic event. Unfortunately, the CT does not give much further information about the age of the lesion or its possible aetiology, which might be helpful in deciding on how to manage this patient further.

2. What further information is needed to guide decision-making with respect to thrombolysis?

The first decision that has to be made is whether or not this patient has had a stroke. The history may give helpful hints here. If possible, the exact symptom onset should be elucidated. Was it sudden or did it occur over some minutes, which might favour migraine. Were there any abnormal movements at the start, which could indicate a focal motor seizure with subsequent Todd's palsy? Are previous notes available, which may sometimes give more detailed evidence of previous events? Of course, the patient's blood sugar should be checked to rule out hypoglycaemia. Physical examination may give further hints, for example regarding the organicity of the patient's symptoms.

If, with all of this information available, the decision is that the patient's current symptoms are due to ischaemia, the next question is whether he has any contraindications to thrombolysis. While symptom onset 90 minutes earlier would make him a candidate, the presence of a possibly recent ischaemic lesion on CT would be a contraindication. If available, the patient should undergo MRI with DWI sequences, which would be highly likely to show any acute ischaemic lesion. MRI may also be helpful in determining the aetiology and age of the lesion seen on CT. Even if not responsible for the current symptoms, it may still be related to the current event in that there may have been asymptomatic ischaemia due to the same aetiology some days or weeks previously. The presence of a subacute ischaemic lesion would greatly aid the decision as to whether thrombolysis is indicated in this patient, as a stroke in the 3 months prior to the presenting event would be a contraindication. If MRI is unavailable, CT perfusion imaging may also help in establishing any ischaemic areas in the brain. Finally, vascular imaging with MRA or CTA might show the aetiology of the stroke (e.g. a vascular dissection).

It may be difficult to get all of this information within the time window for thrombolysis, and a degree of uncertainty may well remain. The aim in this patient has to be to decide whether he has had a stroke, and if he has any clear contraindications to thrombolysis. The decision whether to thrombolyse then depends on the balance of potential benefits, i.e. the severity of the patient's current deficit, versus the potential risks, i.e. the risk of haemorrhage in the probable presence of an infarct of currently undetermined age.

Case 51.C

An 80-year-old man developed a sudden onset of weakness in the left leg, resulting in a fall. During the fall, he hit his head on a cabinet and sustained right frontal bruising. He denied losing consciousness at any point. On examination, he had a haematoma over the right frontal region, a dense left hemiparesis, and dysarthria, but his level of consciousness was normal. CT brain showed no evidence of a skull fracture, no subdural bleeding, no intracerebral bleeding, and no early signs of infarction. By the time the CT result was available, it was 2.5 hours since symptom onset.

Question

1. Would you thrombolyse this patient?

Answer

1. Would you thrombolyse this patient?

The possible contraindication to thrombolysis in this patient is the head injury which he sustained during the onset of his stroke. If this patient is thrombolysed, his frontal bruising may enlarge significantly. However, the scalp is not a 'non-compressible site', and enlargement of the bruise could be minimized by, for example, applying a tight bandage. As such, subcutaneous bruising may be cosmetically unpleasant and it may take some time to resolve, but it is unlikely to be dangerous and probably does not represent a contraindication to thrombolysis. More important is the question of whether the fall could have resulted in an intracranial injury, which may lead to an intracranial haematoma if the patient is thrombolysed. The patient is currently alert and orientated. There was no loss of consciousness, there is no skull fracture, and there is no evidence of blood on CT 2.5 hours after the injury. The patient has a significant deficit, which has not improved since symptom onset. Given his age, he may well run into further complications from his stroke (e.g. pneumonia) if his hemiparesis renders him bedbound. He potentially has a lot to gain from thrombolysis, the head injury does not appear to be significant, and any bleeding into the subcutaneous bruising can be controlled. While the head injury adds a degree of uncertainty, it is not a clear contraindication, and in this patient the potential benefits of thrombolysis probably outweigh the risks.

Case 51.D

A 75-year-old woman presented with a 1 hour history of sudden onset of right-sided weakness (face, arm) and dysphasia. She had a history of hypertension and osteoarthritis. She was taking aspirin, amlodipine, and bendroflumethiazide. On examination, pulse was 80bpm regular, blood pressure was 190/120mm/Hg, and there was right facial weakness, right arm weakness, and severe global dysphasia. CT brain showed some changes consistent with white matter disease, with hypodense changes around the temporal horns.

Questions

1. Would you thrombolyse this patient?
2. Would you treat her blood pressure?

Answers

1. Would you thrombolyse this patient?

This patient has a severe neurological deficit, she presented very early, and she stands to gain considerably from recanalization. However, at this moment her blood pressure is too high to administer thrombolysis safely. Furthermore, her small vessel disease may increase her risk of haemorrhage with thrombolysis, particularly if this is also associated with the presence of microhaemorrhages (see Case 41). However, these are only visible on gradient echo MRI, and while white matter disease may increase the risk of haemorrhage, it is not a contraindication to thrombolysis.

2. Would you treat her blood pressure?

Treatment of hypertension in acute stroke is a much debated issue. The elevated blood pressure may be a response of the brain to ischaemia, and an attempt to ensure adequate perfusion. Lowering blood pressure may result in hypoperfusion and further ischaemic injury. Generally, hypertension in stroke is managed by looking for and managing possible underlying causes, such as pain, anxiety, or a full bladder. High blood pressure is not usually treated acutely with medication unless it produces symptoms, such as hypertensive encephalopathy.

This approach changes if a patient is a possible candidate for thrombolysis, as is the current case. In this woman, the high blood pressure is the only contraindication to thrombolysis. She presented early, and therefore it may be possible to control her blood pressure while still in the time window for administering TPA. Guidelines for thrombolysis state a cut-off for giving TPA as a blood pressure ≥185/110mmHg. This patient is not too far from this. Her blood pressure may settle spontaneously, and it may be sufficient to re-measure it after 5–10 minutes. If it does not go below 185/110mmHg, it would be appropriate to lower it carefully, for example by giving 10mg labetalol IV injected slowly over 5–10 minutes or with a glyceryl trinitrate infusion. In patients who receive thrombolysis, blood pressure should be lowered to below 185/110mmHg prior to initiating therapy, and it should be kept below this level for 24 hours following thrombolysis.

Case 51.E

An 85-year-old woman with known rheumatoid arthritis and cognitive impairment presented to the emergency department with a 1 hour history of left face, arm, and leg weakness. She was normally wheelchair bound and required assistance from her husband and once-daily carers for dressing and washing. She was taking methotrexate, thyroxine, laxatives, paracetamol, codeine phosphate, citalopram, and Ca and bisphophonates. CT brain showed moderate involutional changes and extensive white matter disease.

Question

1. Would you thrombolyse this patient?

Answer

1. Would you thrombolyse this patient?

This woman has very probably had an ischaemic stroke. She is well within the time frame for thrombolysis, and there are no absolute contraindications for thrombolysing her. Nevertheless, there are a number of issues which increase the risk of thrombolysis, and overall the risk–benefit ratio may not be favourable enough to warrant this treatment and its risks.

First, this woman is already severely disabled and wheelchair bound from her rheumatoid arthritis. Therefore it can be argued that any benefits from thrombolysis may not be particularly great.

The patient also has cognitive impairment and may not be able to grasp the potential risks and benefits of thrombolysis and consent to this treatment. Of course, this can be discussed with the family, who may be able to advise on her attitudes, but it is uncertain if thrombolysis would be in this patient's best interest.

In Europe, thrombolysis is not recommended in patients over the age of 80 years. However, there is some evidence that elderly patients do benefit, and further studies are ongoing, so this is probably only a relative contraindication.

Clinically the patient presents with a lacunar syndrome, and her CT brain shows extensive white matter disease. This patient's symptoms are very likely due to a lacunar stroke. There is some evidence that patients with lacunar stroke benefit less from thrombolysis.

Patients with white matter disease often also have cerebral microbleeds; however, these only show up on MRI. Nevertheless, there is some evidence that the risk of cerebral haemorrhage after thrombolysis is higher in patients with white matter disease, and therefore may be higher in this patient.

Overall, while there are no definite contraindications to thrombolysis in this woman, her chances of benefit are probably reduced because of her significant pre-existing disability, her cognitive impairment, and the likely lacunar stroke. Nevertheless, recanalization with resolution of the hemiparesis may prevent potentially life-threatening complications of a stroke, such as pneumonia. Conversely, the risks of thrombolysis may be increased in this patient because of her advanced age and the extensive small vessel disease, and an ICH as a complication of thrombolysis could be fatal. The cognitive impairment will make it difficult or impossible to discuss these issues with her meaningfully. Thrombolysis may not be in her best interest and the decision whether to proceed should, if possible, be made after discussion with the family, who may be able to indicate if the patient would be willing to take the risk. This case shows that, even if guidelines are followed, the decision whether to thrombolyse is not always straightforward, and that many other factors have to be taken into account to decide on an individual patient's potential risks and benefits of treatment.

Case 51.F

A 63-year-old librarian underwent a coronary artery bypass graft (CABG) for triple vessel disease discovered on routine angiography for exercise-induced angina. He had a past history of severe osteoarthritis and had had a road traffic accident some years previously resulting in a right leg deformity. Two weeks after surgery, he underwent angiography after an equivocal bicycle exercise tolerance test. Whilst in the angiography laboratory, he suddenly stopped speaking and developed a dense right-sided weakness.

Questions

1. What has happened? Describe the likely aetiology and possible mechanisms for this patient's symptoms.
2. How frequently does this complication occur?
3. Would you thrombolyse this patient? Which options would you consider?

Answers

1. What has happened? Describe the likely aetiology and possible mechanisms for this patient's symptoms.

Clinically, this patient appears to have had a large ischaemic event in the left MCA territory. The most likely aetiology is embolization caused by the coronary angiography. This can be caused by dislodging atherosclerotic material from the vessel wall, by thrombus formation and embolization from the angiography catheter, by direct arterial injury with subsequent thrombus formation and embolization, or by an air embolus.

2. How frequently does this complication occur?

Stroke as a consequence of coronary angiography is a serious but rare complication. It occurs in less than 0.5% of patients (*Circulation* 1976). More studies are available for percutaneous coronary angioplasty or stenting, and stroke has been reported to occur in 0.07–0.3% of all percutaneous coronary interventions.

3. Would you thrombolyse this patient? Which options would you consider?

This patient has probably had an iatrogenic embolization to his left MCA. Symptom onset appears to have been a few minutes earlier, and so he would be well within the time window for thrombolysis. Both IV thrombolysis and intra-arterial recanalization are therapeutic options.

The patient has two possible contraindications to IV thrombolysis according to the guidelines of the American Stroke Association which recommend avoiding IV thrombolysis within 14 days after major surgery. The patient had had a CABG 2 weeks earlier, so his recent surgery is a relative contraindication to thrombolysis, although the patient is only just still within this time window. The guidelines also recommend that IV thrombolysis should not be carried out within 3 months of a myocardial infarction. This is because of the risk of causing myocardial rupture. Although the patient has had coronary surgery, this would not usually cause significant myocardial damage, and there is no history of myocardial infarction, so this risk is probably not significantly increased and would not represent a contraindication to thrombolysis.

The extent of the patient's neurological deficit and the probable embolic origin of his stroke make it very likely that he has a large vessel occlusion, probably affecting either the main stem or major branches of the MCA. Recanalization of embolic large vessel occlusions can be difficult to achieve with IV thrombolysis, which may reduce the chances of a good outcome in this setting.

Even though its benefits have not yet been clearly established, an endovascular approach to recanalization should be considered in this patient, given that he is in hospital and even already in the angiography suite. Treatment options include intra-arterial thrombolysis, or the use of a mechanical thrombectomy device if a neuroradiology service with the appropriate experience is available. Several studies have shown that intra-arterial thrombolysis or mechanical clot disruption or retrieval improve vascular recanalization rates compared with IV thrombolysis, although there is no clear evidence that this also leads to a better clinical outcome. Nevertheless, as there is a high chance of this patient having a large vessel occlusion, his chances of recanalization are probably higher with intra-arterial intervention rather than IV thrombolysis. He is already in the angiography suite, so the frequent argument that intra-arterial treatment takes longer to set up and increases the time from symptom onset to treatment should not apply. An intra-arterial approach would also reduce the amount of thrombolytic agent in the systemic circulation, which, in view of his recent surgery, may reduce the risk of haemorrhage compared with IV thrombolysis.

It has been found in several case series that intra-arterial thrombolysis and/or mechanical recanalization can be achieved successfully and safely in patients with stroke after angiography. If the facilities exist, this would also be a reasonable approach in this patient. He should have a cerebral angiogram and if this confirms a large vessel occlusion, intra-arterial thrombolysis or endovascular recanalization should be considered. If these facilities are not available, one has to weigh the risks of IV thrombolysis causing a possibly fatal haemorrhage 2 weeks after coronary surgery against the potential benefit of avoiding a severely disabling neurological deficit. As patients may already be anticoagulated 48 hours after CABG (e.g. if they develop AF), one might expect thrombolysis 2 weeks after surgery to be reasonably safe. Given that the patient is at high risk of remaining severely disabled if his vessel does not recanalize, IV thrombolysis appears to be a reasonable treatment if intra-arterial intervention is not available. However, intra-arterial intervention in this patient may be preferable, because of both the likely lower interventional risk and the higher chance of achieving recanalization.

Case 51.G

A 70-year-old woman presented with right face, arm, and leg weakness, gaze deviation to the left, and global aphasia. The family gave a history of onset 1 hour and 20 minutes previously. There was a past history of hypertension and non-ST elevation myocardial infarction. Medication included aspirin, simvastatin, lisinopril, and bisoprolol. Blood tests and CT brain scan were unremarkable, and thrombolysis was instituted. Ten minutes later, the left side of the patient's tongue began to swell, followed by the rest of her tongue and her neck. The intensive care team was called and nasal intubation was instituted. Intramuscular adrenaline, IV antihistamine, and steroids were administered. The patient eventually made a good recovery, both from her acute deterioration and from her neurological deficits.

Questions

1. What condition has this patient developed?
2. Is the medication history relevant?
3. What should have been done prior to institution of thrombolytic therapy?
4. Would you have managed the tongue swelling differently?

Answers

1. What condition has this patient developed?

The patient has developed orolingual angio-oedema. This is a recognized side effect of treatment with TPA, and occurs in approximately 1–2% of thrombolysed stroke patients. The probable mechanism is the conversion of plasminogen to plasmin by TPA. Plasmin activates the complement cascade, especially C1 and C3, which leads to the degranulation of mast cells with histamine release and vasodilation. Furthermore, plasmin also promotes the conversion of kininogen to bradykinin, which again causes vasodilation, plasma extravasation, and mucosal oedema. The incidence of angio-oedema appears to be higher in stroke than after thrombolysis for myocardial infarction. This may be due to autonomic dysfunction caused by cerebral ischaemia, which increases the tendency to develop angio-oedema. The presence of ischaemic injury may also explain why angio-oedema is often unilateral, occurring on the contralateral side of the infarct. Ischaemic injury affecting the contralateral insular cortex appears to be particularly frequent in patients who develop angio-oedema after thrombolysis for stroke.

2. Is the medication history relevant?

The patient has a history of hypertension which is treated with lisinopril. Patients who take ACE inhibitors appear to be more likely to develop angio-oedema. ACE inhibitors slow down the breakdown of bradykinin, the level of which is increased after administration of TPA. Reduced clearance of bradykinin increases the chances of angio-oedema developing, becoming more severe, and resolving more slowly.

3. What should have been done prior to institution of thrombolytic therapy?

It is important to be aware of the potential risk of angio-oedema with TPA, in particular in patients on ACE inhibitors. A potential differential diagnosis is the development of tongue haematoma, and a patient's mouth should be inspected for injury and tongue bites prior to instituting TPA. To be able to deal with angio-oedema quickly, the relevant medication (steroids and antihistamines) should be available, as should facilities for intubation.

4. Would you have managed the tongue swelling differently?

Treatment of orolingual angio-oedema is directed at reducing the effects of histamines and maintaining the airway. While there is little evidence base, extrapolating from angio-oedema occurring with the administration of ACE inhibitors, the current recommended treatment is to give antihistamines and steroids (e.g. chlorphenamine 10mg IV and hydrocortisone 100–200mg). Intubation may be necessary. The use of adrenaline in this situation is risky, and should probably be avoided if possible as it will lead to peaks in blood pressure which are dangerous and may promote ICH in stroke patients who have been thrombolysed.

Further reading

Adams HP Jr, del Zoppo G, Alberts MJ, *et al.* (2007). Guidelines for the early management of adults with ischemic stroke. *Stroke*; **38**: 1655–1711.

Appelboom G, Strozyk D, Meyers PM, Higashida RT (2010). Current recommendations for endovascular interventions in the treatment of ischemic stroke. *Curr Atheroscler Rep*; **12**: 244–50.

Arnold M, Fischer U, Schroth G, *et al.* (2008). Intra-arterial thrombolysis of acute iatrogenic intracranial arterial occlusion attributable to neuroendovascular procedures or coronary angiography. *Stroke*; **39**: 1491–5.

Engelter ST, Fluri F, Buitrago-Tellez C, *et al.* (2005). Life-threatening orolingual angioedema during thrombolysis in acute ischemic stroke. *J Neurol*; **22**: 1167–70.

Tomsick TA, Khatri P, Jovin T, *et al.* (2010). Equipoise among recanalisation strategies. *Neurology*; **74**: 1069–76.

World Stroke Academy. *Learning Module Hyperacute Stroke.* http://www.world-stroke-academy.org/online_learning_hyperacute.php.

List of cases by diagnosis

Case 1: Brain tumour mimicking stroke
Case 2: Stroke mimicking brain tumour
Case 3: Lateral medullary syndrome
Case 4: Multiple strokes from atrial fibrillation and undiagnosed mitral valve disease
Case 5: Homocystinuria
Case 6: Cerebral amyloid angiopathy
Case 7: Migraine
Case 8: Post-stroke dementia
Case 9: Bickerstaff's encephalitis
Case 10: Bilateral hemisphere symptoms and difficult endarterectomy decision
Case 11: Varicella zoster vasculopathy
Case 12: Transient ischaemic attack thought to be non-organic symptoms
Case 13: Demyelination
Case 14: Cerebellar stroke
Case 15: Giant cell arteritis
Case 16: Anatomical variants of cerebral vasculature
Case 17: Venous sinus thrombosis and ear infection
Case 18: Transient global amnesia
Case 19: Carotid disease
Case 20: Conversion disorder
Case 21: Asymptomatic cerebral aneurysm
Case 22: Occult atrial fibrillation
Case 23: Partial seizure
Case 24: Traumatic ICA-dissection and hemicraniectomy after malignant MCA infarction
Case 25: Systemic lupus erythematosus
Case 26: Peripheral nerve disorder
Case 27: Differential diagnosis of dysarthria
Case 28: CADASIL
Case 29: Diplopia
Case 30: Recurrent haemorrhage into tumour
Case 31: Intracranial atheroma
Case 32: Severe carotid stenosis and multiple infarctions
Case 33: Creutzfeldt–Jakob disease
Case 34: Reversible cerebral vasoconstriction syndrome
Case 35: Amaurosis fugax
Case 36: Fibromuscular dysplasia
Case 37: Cardiac tumour
Case 38: Limb-shaking (low-flow) transient ischaemic attack
Case 39: Cerebral abscess
Case 40: Moyamoya disease
Case 41: Inflammatory bowel disease, paroxysmal atrial fibrillation, and microbleeds
Case 42: Todd's paresis
Case 43: Delirium
Case 44: Cavernoma

List of cases by clinical features

Stroke/TIA mimics: *1, 7, 9, 13, 18, 20, 23, 26, 29, 33, 39, 42*
Haemorrhage: *6, 30, 46, 47, 51*
Small vessel disease: *8, 22, 28, 37, 41, 43, 45, 49*
Large vessel disease: *3, 10, 14, 19, 31, 32*
Cardiac disease: *4, 22, 37, 41, 47, 48*
Recurrent/multiple stroke: *4, 6, 8, 10, 11, 15, 22, 25, 28, 30, 32, 45, 47, 50*
Microbleeds: *6, 28, 41*
Vasculitis/angiopathy: *6, 11, 15, 25, 28, 34, 36, 40, 50*
Low flow: *15, 38, 40*
Encephalopathy: *4, 9, 24, 25, 34, 39, 43, 50*
Memory/cognitive disturbance: *6, 8, 18, 28, 33, 43, 49*
Infection: *11, 17, 39, 47*
Endarterectomy/endovascular intervention/neurosurgery: *3, 10, 14, 19, 21, 24, 46, 48*
DWI in diagnosis/management: *4, 10, 25, 32, 39, 43, 50*
Seizures: *6, 23, 25, 42*

Index